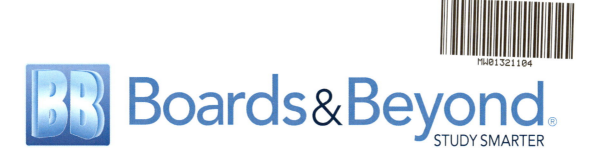

Boards & Beyond: Biochemistry Slides

Color slides for USMLE Step 1 preparation
from the Boards and Beyond Website

Jason Ryan, MD, MPH

2022 Edition

Boards & Beyond provides a virtual medical school curriculm used by students around the globe to supplement their education and prepare for board exams such as USMLE Step 1.

This book of slides is intended as a companion to the videos for easy reference and note-taking. Videos are subject to change without notice. PDF versions of all color books are available via the website as part of membership.

Visit www.boardsbeyond.com to learn more.

Copyright © 2022 Boards and Beyond
All rights reserved.

Table of Contents

DNA Structure 1	Ethanol Metabolism 63
Purine Metabolism 5	Exercise and Starvation 67
Pyrimidine Metabolism 10	Inborn Errors of Metabolism 73
Glucose 16	Amino Acids 78
Glycolysis 19	Phenylalanine and Tyrosine 82
Gluconeogenesis 25	Other Amino Acids 89
Glycogen 29	Ammonia 95
HMP Shunt 34	B Vitamins 101
Fructose and Galactose 38	Folate and Vitamin B12 109
Pyruvate Dehydrogenase 42	Other Vitamins 113
TCA Cycle 46	Lipid Metabolism 121
Electron Transport Chain 50	Hyperlipidemia 127
Fatty Acids 55	Lipid Drugs 130
Ketone Bodies 61	Lysosomal Storage Diseases 136

DNA Structure

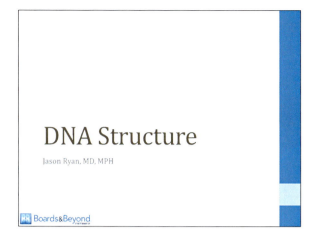

DNA Structure
Jason Ryan, MD, MPH

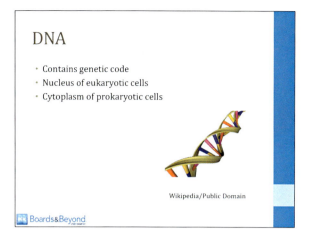

DNA
- Contains genetic code
- Nucleus of eukaryotic cells
- Cytoplasm of prokaryotic cells

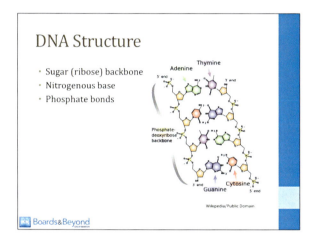

DNA Structure
- Sugar (ribose) backbone
- Nitrogenous base
- Phosphate bonds

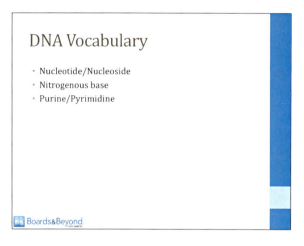

DNA Vocabulary
- Nucleotide/Nucleoside
- Nitrogenous base
- Purine/Pyrimidine

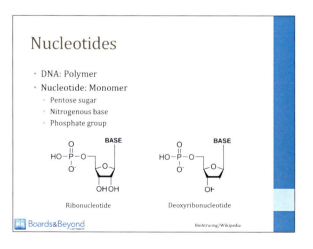

Nucleotides
- DNA: Polymer
- Nucleotide: Monomer
  - Pentose sugar
  - Nitrogenous base
  - Phosphate group

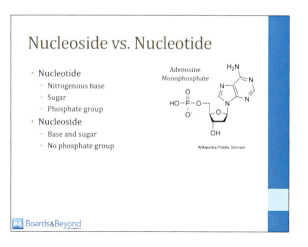

Nucleoside vs. Nucleotide
- Nucleotide
  - Nitrogenous base
  - Sugar
  - Phosphate group
- Nucleoside
  - Base and sugar
  - No phosphate group

Adenosine Monophosphate

Nitrogenous Bases

Pyrimidines: Cytosine, Thymine, Uracil

Purines: Adenine, Guanine

Nucleotides

Cytidine, Thymidine, Uridine, Adenosine, Guanosine

Nucleotides

- Synthesized as monophosphates
- Converted to triphosphate form
- Added to DNA

Deoxyadenosine Triphosphate

Base Pairing

- DNA
  - Adenine-Thymine
  - Guanine-Cytosine
- RNA
  - Adenine-Uracil
  - Guanine-Cytosine

More C-G bonds = ↑ Melting temperature

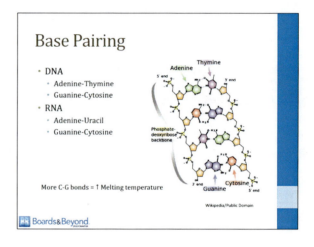

DNA Methylation

- Methyl group added to cytosine
  - Occurs in segments with CG patterns ("CG islands")
  - Both strands
- Inactivates transcription ("epigenetics")
- Human DNA: ~70% methylated
- Unmethylated CG stimulate immune response

Cytosine → 5-methylcytosine

Bacterial DNA Methylation

- Bacteria methylate cytosine and adenine
- Methylation protects bacteria from viruses (phages)
- Non-methylated DNA destroyed by endonucleases
- "Restriction-modification systems"

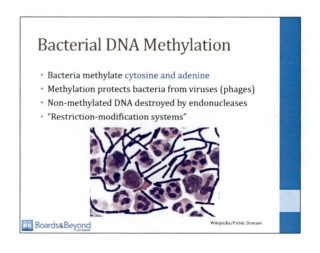

Chromatin

- Found in nucleus of eukaryotic cells
- DNA plus proteins = chromatin
- Chromatin condenses into chromosomes

Nucleosome

- Key protein: Histones
- Units of histones plus DNA = nucleosomes

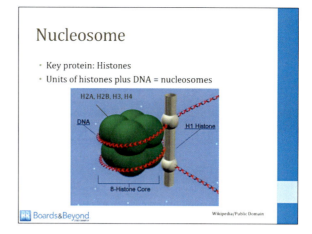

Histones

- Peptides
  - H1, H2A, H2B, H3, H4
- Contain **basic** amino acids
  - High content of lysine, arginine
  - Positively charged
  - Binds negatively charged phosphate backbone
- H1 distinct from others
  - Not in nucleosome core
  - Larger, more basic
  - Ties beads on string together

DNA Structure

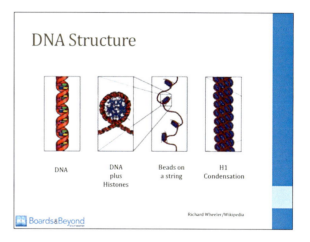

DNA | DNA plus Histones | Beads on a string | H1 Condensation

Drug-Induced Lupus

- Fever, joint pains, rash after starting drug
- Anti-histone antibodies (>95% cases)
  - Contrast with anti-dsDNA in classic lupus
- Classic drugs:
  - Hydralazine
  - Procainamide
  - Isoniazid

Chromatin Types

- Heterochromatin
  - Condensed
  - Gene sequences not transcribed (varies by cell)
  - Significant DNA methylation
- Euchromatin
  - Less condensed
  - Transcription
  - Significant histone acetylation

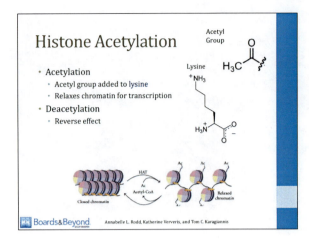

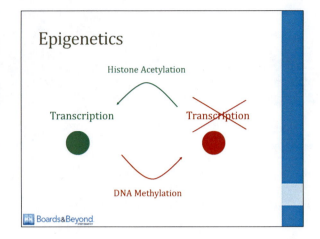

Histone deacetylase inhibitors
HDACs

- Potential therapeutic effects
- Anti-cancer
  - Increased expression of HDACs some tumors
- Huntington's disease
  - Movement disorder
  - Abnormal huntingtin protein
  - Gain of function mutation (mutant protein)
  - Possible mechanism: histone deacetylation → gene silencing
  - Leads to neuronal cell death in striatum

Dokmanovic et al. **Histone deacetylase inhibitors: overview and perspectives**
Mol Cancer Res. 2007 Oct;5(10):981-9.

Purine Metabolism

Purine Metabolism
Jason Ryan, MD, MPH

Nucleotides

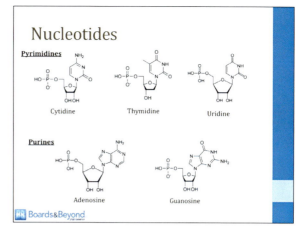

Pyrimidines: Cytidine, Thymidine, Uridine
Purines: Adenosine, Guanosine

Nucleotide Roles

- RNA and DNA monomers
- Energy: ATP
- Physiologic mediators
  - cAMP levels → blood flow
  - cGMP → second messenger

Sources of Nucleotides

- Diet (exogenous)
- Biochemical synthesis (endogenous)
  - Direct synthesis
  - Salvage

Key Points

- Ribonucleic acids (RNA) synthesized first
- RNA converted to *deoxy*ribonucleic acids (DNA)
- Different pathways for purines versus pyrimidines
- All nitrogen comes from **amino acids**

Purine Synthesis

- Goal is to create AMP and GMP
- Ingredients:
  - Ribose phosphate (HMP Shunt)
  - Amino acids
  - Carbons (tetrahydrofolate, CO_2)

Adenosine, Guanosine

Purine Synthesis

- Step 1: Create **PRPP**

Ribose 5-phosphate → 5-Phosphoribosyl-1-pyrophosphate (PRPP)

Purine Synthesis

- Step 2: Create **IMP**

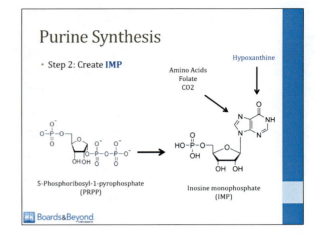

5-Phosphoribosyl-1-pyrophosphate (PRPP) → Inosine monophosphate (IMP)

Amino Acids, Folate, CO2, Hypoxanthine

Purine Synthesis

- Two rings with two nitrogens:
  - 6 unit, 3 double bonds
  - 5 unit, 2 double bonds

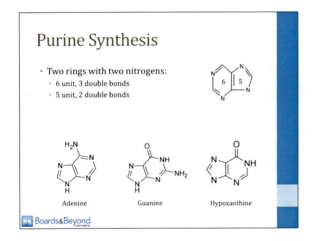

Adenine, Guanine, Hypoxanthine

Purine Synthesis
Nitrogen Sources

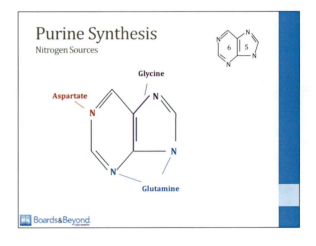

Aspartate, Glycine, Glutamine

Purine Synthesis
Carbon Sources

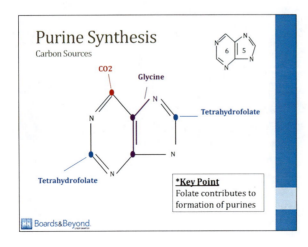

CO2, Glycine, Tetrahydrofolate, Tetrahydrofolate

*Key Point
Folate contributes to formation of purines

Purine Synthesis

- Step 3: Create AMP and GMP

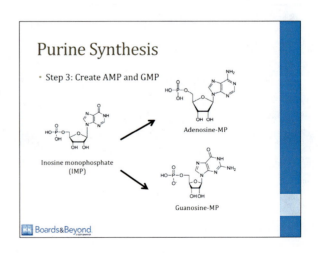

Inosine monophosphate (IMP) → Adenosine-MP, Guanosine-MP

Purine Synthesis
Summary

- Starts with ribose phosphate from HMP shunt
- Key intermediates are **PRPP** and **IMP**

5-Ribose Phosphate → PRPP → IMP → AMP / GMP

(Aspartate, Glycine, Glutamine, THF, CO_2)

Purine Synthesis
Regulation

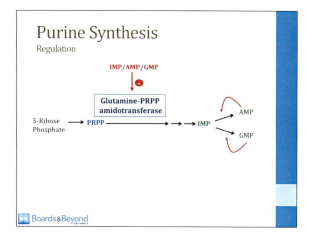

Deoxyribonucleotides

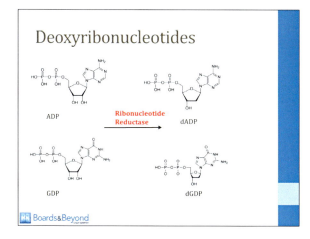

ADP → dADP (Ribonucleotide Reductase)
GDP → dGDP

Purine Synthesis
Drugs & Diseases

- Ribavirin (antiviral)
  - Inhibits IMP dehydrogenase
  - Blocks conversion IMP to GMP
  - Inhibits synthesis guanine nucleotides (purines)
- Mycophenolate (immunosuppressant)
  - Inhibits IMP dehydrogenase

Purine Fates

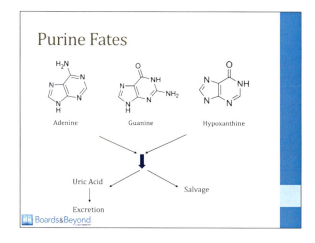

Adenine, Guanine, Hypoxanthine → Uric Acid → Excretion / Salvage

Purine Salvage

- Salvages bases: adenine, guanine, hypoxanthine
- Converts back into nucleotides: AMP, GMP, IMP
- Requires PRPP

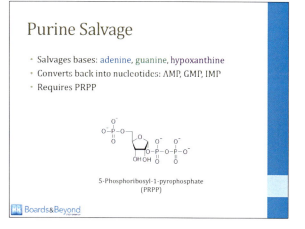

5-Phosphoribosyl-1-pyrophosphate (PRPP)

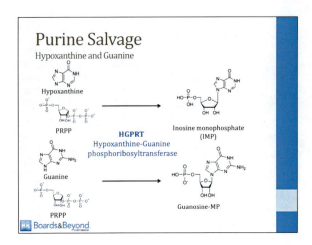
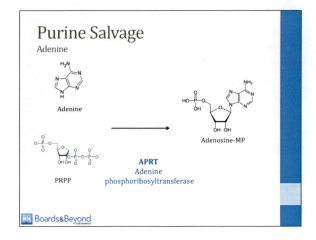
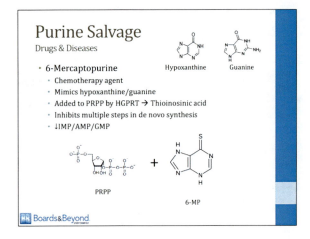
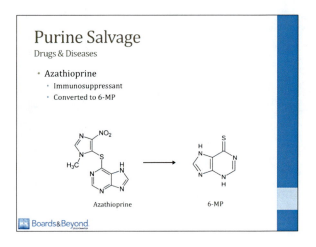
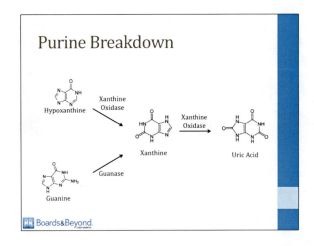
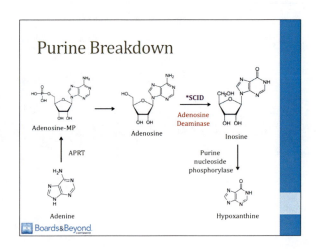

Purine Salvage
Drugs & Diseases

- Gout
  - Excess uric acid
  - Crystal deposition in joints → pain, swelling, redness
  - Can occur from overproduction of uric acid
  - High cell turnover (trauma, chemotherapy)
  - Consumption of purine-rich foods (**meat**, **seafood**)
  - Treatment: inhibit xanthine oxidase (**allopurinol**)

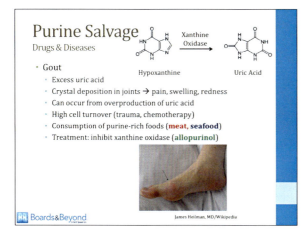

Hypoxanthine → (Xanthine Oxidase) → Uric Acid

James Heilman, MD/Wikipedia

Purine Salvage
Drugs & Diseases

- Azathioprine and 6-MP
  - Metabolized by **xanthine oxidase**
  - Caution with allopurinol
  - May boost effects
  - May increase toxicity

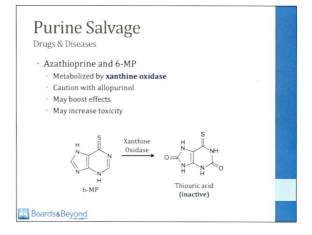

6-MP → (Xanthine Oxidase) → Thiouric acid (**inactive**)

Purine Salvage
Drugs & Diseases

- Lesch-Nyhan syndrome
  - **X-linked absence of HGPRT**
  - **Excess uric acid** production ("juvenile gout")
  - Excess de novo purine synthesis (↑**PRPP**, ↑**IMP**)
  - Neurologic impairment (mechanism unclear)
  - Hypotonia, chorea
  - Classic feature: self mutilating behavior (biting, scratching)
  - Can treat hyperuricemia
  - Limited treatments for neurologic features
- Classic presentation
  - Male child with motor symptoms, self-mutilation, gout

Purine Metabolism
Summary

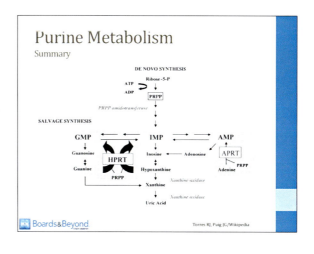

Torres RJ, Puig JG/Wikipedia

Pyrimidine Metabolism

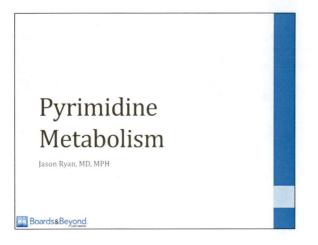

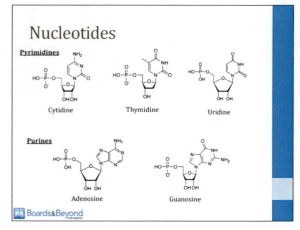

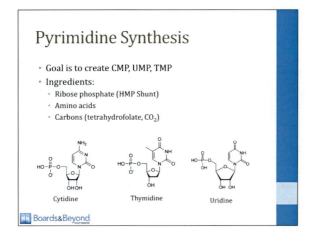

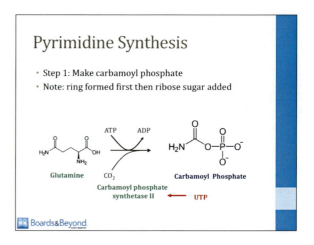

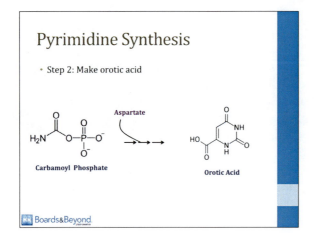

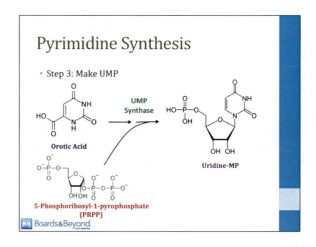

Key Point

- UMP synthesized first
- CMP, TMP derived from UMP

Glutamine → Carbamoyl Phosphate → Orotic Acid → UMP → CMP / TMP

UMP Synthase
Bifunctional

Pyrimidine Ring
Two nitrogens/four carbons

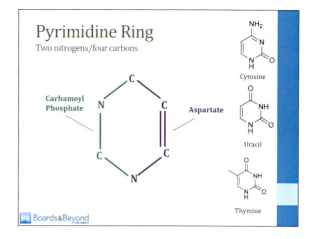

Pyrimidine Synthesis
Drugs and Diseases

- **Orotic aciduria**
  - Autosomal recessive
  - Defect in **UMP synthase**
  - Buildup of orotic acid
  - Loss of pyrimidines

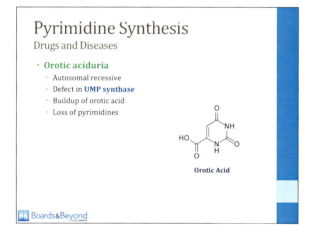

Orotic Acid

Pyrimidine Synthesis
Drugs and Diseases

- Key findings
  - Orotic acid in urine
  - Megaloblastic anemia
  - No B12/folate response
  - Growth retardation
- Treatment:
  - Uridine
  - Bypasses UMP synthase

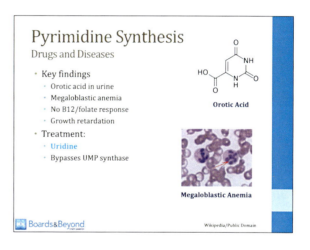

Orotic Acid

Megaloblastic Anemia

Ornithine transcarbamylase
OTC

- Key urea cycle enzyme
- Combines **carbamoyl phosphate** with ornithine
- Makes citrulline
- OTC deficiency → increased **carbamoyl phosphate**
- ↑ carbamoyl phosphate → ↑ orotic acid
- Don't confuse with orotic aciduria
  - Both have orotic aciduria
  - OTC only: ↑ **ammonia levels** (urea cycle dysfunction)
  - Ammonia → encephalopathy (baby with lethargy, coma)

Cytidine

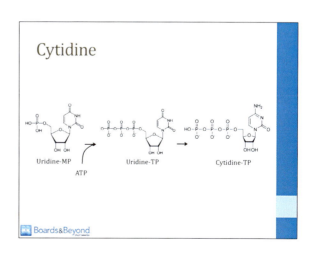

Uridine-MP → Uridine-TP → Cytidine-TP

ATP

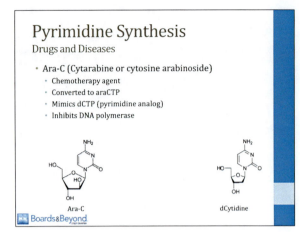

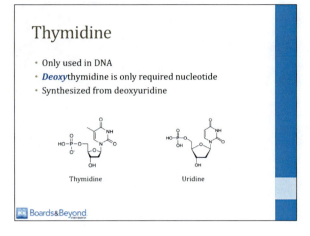

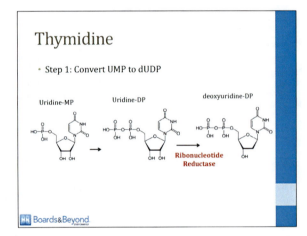

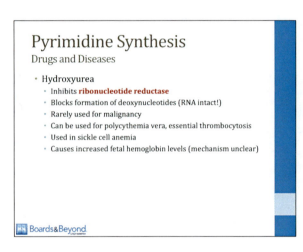

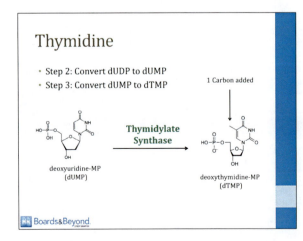

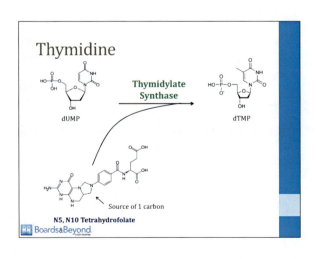

Folate Compounds

Folate

Dihydrofolate

Tetrahydrofolate

Folate Compounds

Tetrahydrofolate

N5, N10 Tetrahydrofolate

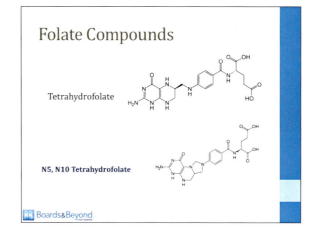

Thymidine

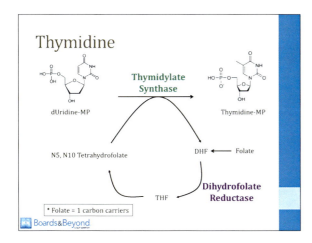

* Folate = 1 carbon carriers

Pyrimidine Synthesis
Drugs and Diseases

- 5-FU
  - Chemotherapy agent
  - Mimics uracil
  - Converted to 5-FdUMP (abnormal dUMP)
  - Covalently binds N5,N10 TFH and thymidylate synthase
  - Result: inhibition thymidylate synthase
  - Blocks dTMP synthesis ("thymineless death")

Uracil

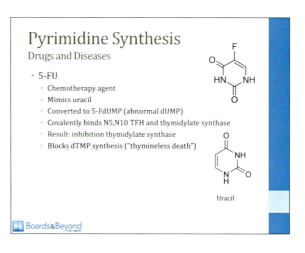

Pyrimidine Synthesis
Drugs and Diseases

- Methotrexate
  - Chemotherapy agent, immunosuppressant
  - Mimics DHF
  - Inhibits dihydrofolate reductase
  - Blocks synthesis dTMP
  - Rescue with leucovorin (folinic acid; converted to THF)

Folate   Methotrexate

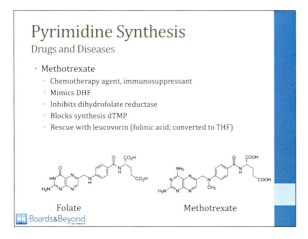

Pyrimidine Synthesis
Drugs and Diseases

- Sulfonamides antibiotics
  - Bacteria cannot absorb folic acid
  - Synthesize THF from para-aminobenzoic acid (PABA)
  - Sulfonamides mimic PABA
  - Block THF synthesis
  - ↓ THF formation → ↓ dTMP (loss of DNA synthesis)
  - No effect human cells (dietary folate)

Sulfanilamide   PABA

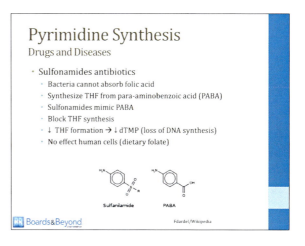

Bacterial THF Synthesis

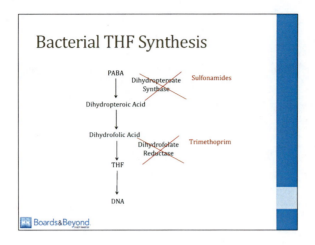

Pyrimidine Synthesis
Drugs and Diseases

- Folate deficiency
  - Main effect: loss of dTMP production → ↓ DNA production
  - RNA production relatively intact (does not require thymidine)
  - **Macrocytic anemia** (fewer but larger RBCs)
  - **Neural tube defects** in pregnancy

Vitamin B12

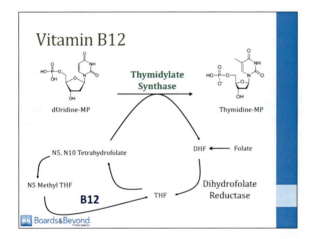

Vitamin B12

- Required to regenerate THF from N5-Methyl THF
- Deficiency = "Methyl folate trap"
- Loss of dTMP synthesis (megaloblastic anemia)
- Neurological dysfunction (demyelination)

Homocysteine and MMA

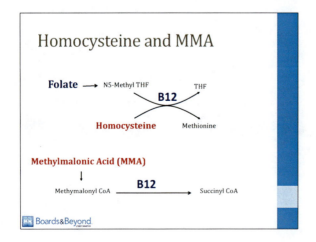

B12 versus Folate Deficiency

- **Homocysteine**
  - Both folate and B12 required to covert to methionine
  - Elevated homocysteine in both deficiencies
- **Methylmalonic Acid**
  - B12 also converts MMA to succinyl CoA
  - B12 deficiency = ↑ methylmalonic acid (MMA) level
  - Folate deficiency = normal MMA level

B12 versus Folate Deficiency

	Folate	B12
RBC	↓	↓
MCV	↑	↑
Homocysteine	↑	↑
Methylmalonic acid (MMA)	--	↑

Megaloblastic Anemia

- Anemia (↓Hct)
- Large RBCs (↑MCV)
- Hypersegmented neutrophils
- Commonly caused by defective DNA production
  - Folate deficiency
  - B12 (neuro symptoms, MMA)
  - Orotic aciduria
  - Drugs (MTX, 5-FU, hydroxyurea)
  - Zidovudine (HIV NRTIs)

Glucose

Glucose

Jason Ryan, MD, MPH

Carbs

- Carbohydrate = "watered carbon"
- Most have formula $C_n(H_2O)_m$

Glucose $C_6H_{12}O_6$

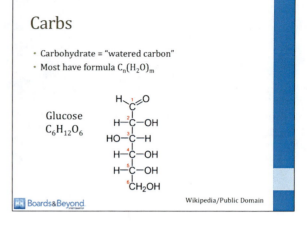

Wikipedia/Public Domain

Carbs

- Monosaccharides ($C_6H_{12}O_6$)
- Glucose, Fructose, Galactose

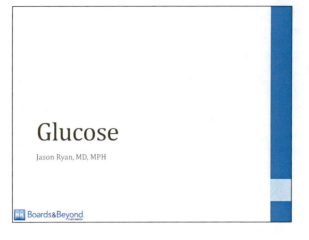

Carbs

- Disaccharides = 2 monosaccharides
- Broken down to monosaccharides in GI tract
- **Lactose** (galactose + glucose); lactase
- **Sucrose** (fructose + glucose); sucrase

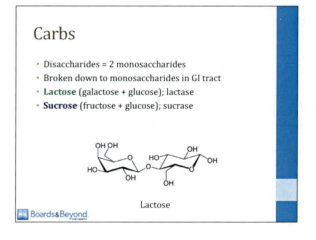

Lactose

Complex Carbs

- Polysaccharides: polymers of monosaccharides
- Starch
  - Plant polysaccharide (glucose polymers)
- Glycogen
  - Animal polysaccharide (also glucose polymers)
- Cellulose
  - Plant polysaccharide of glucose molecules
  - Different bonds from starch
  - Cannot be broken down by animals
  - "Fiber" in diet → improved bowel function

Glucose

- All carbohydrates broken down into:
  - Glucose
  - Fructose
  - Galactose

Glucose Metabolism

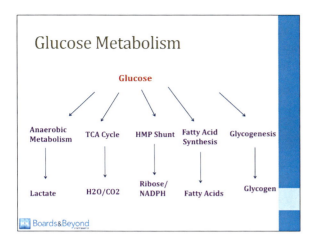

Glucose Metabolism

- Liver
  - Most varied use of glucose
  - TCA cycle for ATP
  - Glycogen synthesis

Glucose Metabolism

- Brain
  - Constant use of glucose for TCA cycle (ATP)
  - Little glycogen storage
- Muscle/heart
  - TCA cycle (ATP)
  - Transport into cells heavily influenced by insulin
  - More insulin → more glucose uptake
  - Store glucose as glycogen

Glucose Metabolism

- Red blood cells
  - No mitochondria
  - Use glucose for anaerobic metabolism (make ATP)
  - Generate lactate
  - Also use glucose for HMP shunt (NADPH)
- Adipose tissue
  - Mostly converts glucose to fatty acids
  - Like muscle, uptake influenced by insulin

Glucose Entry into Cells

- Na+ **independent** entry
  - 14 different transporters described
  - GLUT-1 to GLUT-14
  - Varies by tissue (i.e. GLUT-1 in RBCs)
- Na+ **dependent** entry
  - Glucose absorbed from low → high concentration
  - Intestinal epithelium
  - Renal tubules

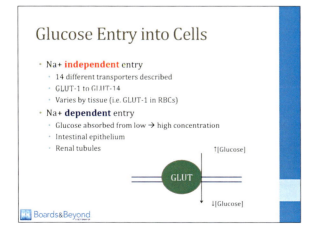

Glucose GI Absorption

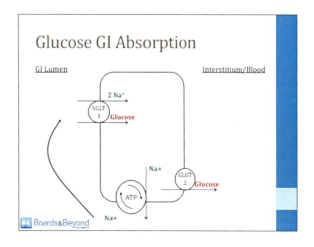

Proximal Tubule

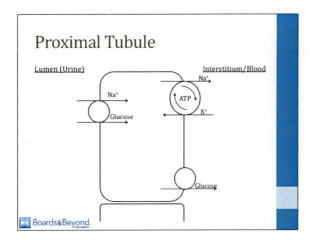

Glucose Entry into Cells

- GLUT-1
  - Insulin **independent** (uptake when [glucose] high)
  - Brain, RBCs
- GLUT-4
  - Insulin **dependent**
  - Fat tissue, skeletal muscle
- GLUT-2
  - Insulin independent
  - **Bidirectional** (gluconeogenesis)
  - Liver, kidney
  - Intestine (glucose OUT of epithelial cells to portal vein)
  - Pancreas

Glycolysis

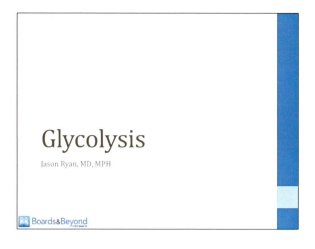

Glycolysis
Jason Ryan, MD, MPH

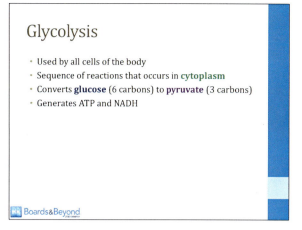

Glycolysis
- Used by all cells of the body
- Sequence of reactions that occurs in **cytoplasm**
- Converts **glucose** (6 carbons) to **pyruvate** (3 carbons)
- Generates ATP and NADH

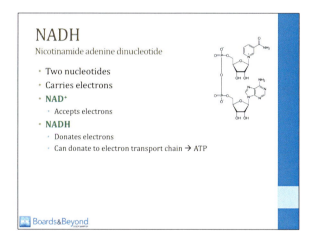

NADH
Nicotinamide adenine dinucleotide

- Two nucleotides
- Carries electrons
- **NAD⁺**
  - Accepts electrons
- **NADH**
  - Donates electrons
  - Can donate to electron transport chain → ATP

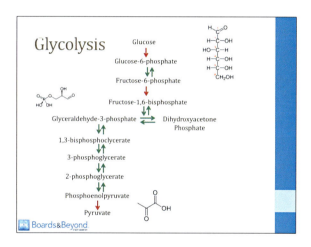

Glycolysis

Glucose
↓
Glucose-6-phosphate
↓↑
Fructose-6-phosphate
↓↑
Fructose-1,6-bisphosphate
↓↑
Glyceraldehyde-3-phosphate ⇌ Dihydroxyacetone Phosphate
↓↑
1,3-bisphosphoglycerate
↓↑
3-phosphoglycerate
↓↑
2-phosphoglycerate
↓↑
Phosphoenolpyruvate
↓
Pyruvate

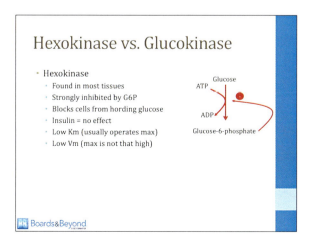

Hexokinase vs. Glucokinase

- Hexokinase
  - Found in most tissues
  - Strongly inhibited by G6P
  - Blocks cells from hording glucose
  - Insulin = no effect
  - Low Km (usually operates max)
  - Low Vm (max is not that high)

Glucose + ATP → Glucose-6-phosphate + ADP

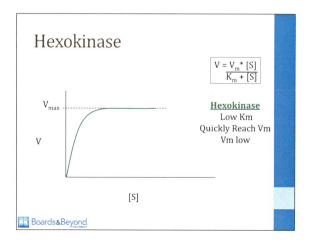

Hexokinase

$$V = \frac{V_m * [S]}{K_m + [S]}$$

Hexokinase
Low Km
Quickly Reach Vm
Vm low

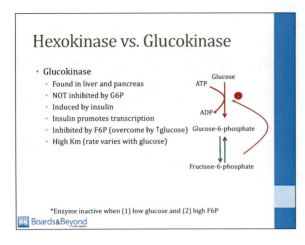
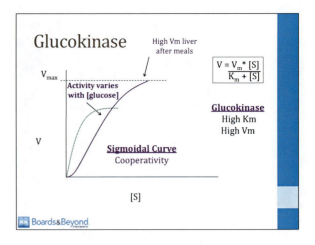
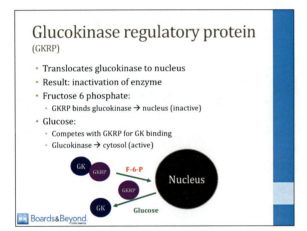
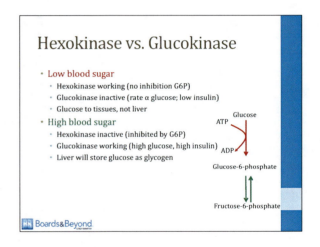
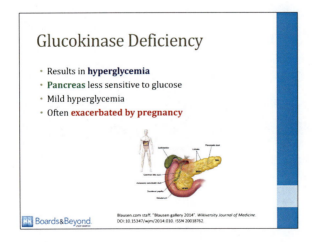
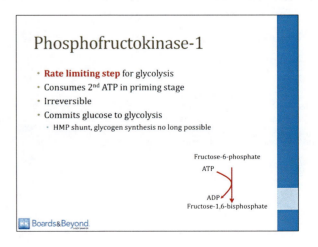

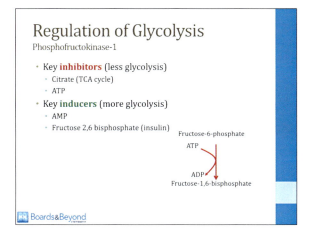
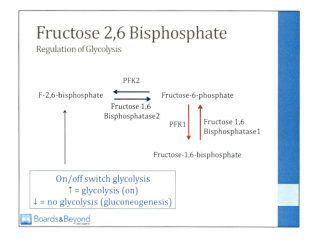
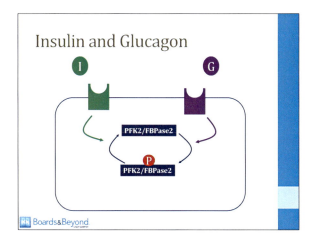
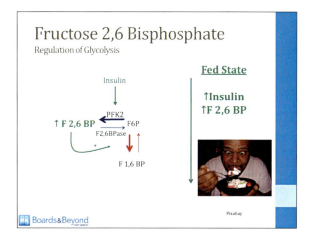
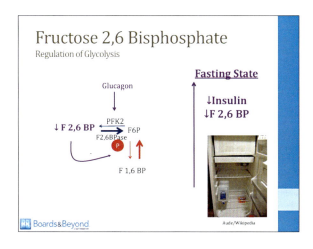
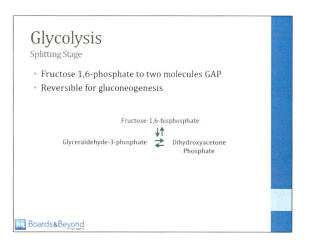

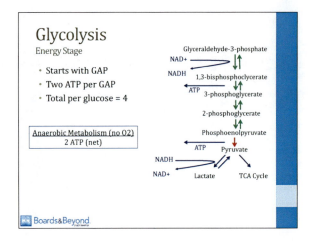
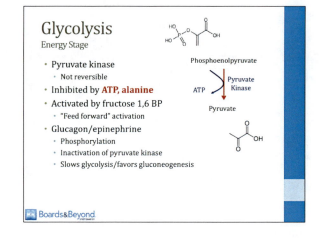
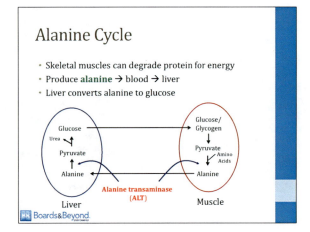
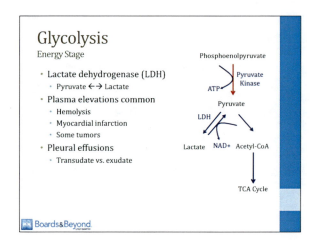
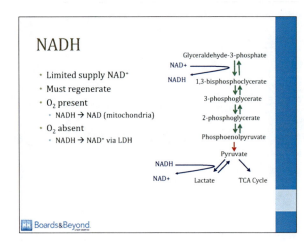
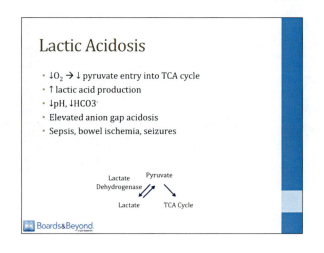

Muscle Cramps

- Too much exercise → too much NAD consumption
  - Exceed capacity of TCA cycle/electron transport
  - Elevated NADH/NAD ratio
- Favors pyruvate → **lactate**
- pH falls in muscles → cramps
- Distance runners: lots of mitochondria (bigger, too)

Pyruvate Kinase Deficiency

- Autosomal recessive disorder
- **RBCs** most effected
  - No mitochondria
  - Require PK for anaerobic metabolism
  - Loss of ATP
  - Membrane failure → phagocytosis in spleen
- Usually presents as **newborn**
- **Extravascular hemolysis**
- Splenomegaly
- Disease severity ranges based on enzyme activity

2,3 Bisphosphoglycerate

- Created from diverted 1,3 BPG
- Used by **RBCs**
  - No mitochondria
  - No TCA cycle
- **Sacrifices ATP** from glycolysis
- 2,3 BPG alters Hgb binding

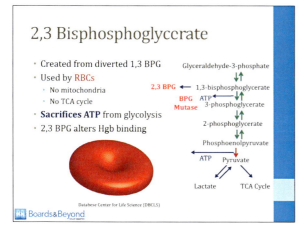

Energy Yield from Glucose

- ATP generated depends on cells/oxygen
- Highest yield with **O_2 and mitochondria**
  - Allows pyruvate to enter TCA cycle
  - Converts pyruvate/NADH → ATP

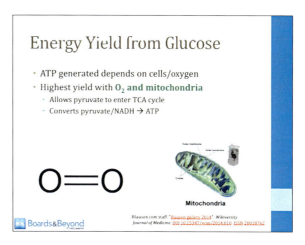

Energy from Glucose

Oxygen and Mitochondria
Glucose + $6O_2$ → **32/30 ATP** + $6CO_2$ + $6 H_2O$
32 ATP = malate-aspartate shuttle (liver, heart)
30 ATP = glycerol-3-phosphate shuttle (muscle)

No Oxygen or No Mitochondria
Glucose → **2 ATP** + 2 Lactate + $2 H_2O$

*RBCs = no mitochondria

Summary
Key Steps

- Regulation
  - #1: Hexokinase/Glucokinase
  - #2: PFK1
  - #3: Pyruvate Kinase
- Irreversible
  - Glucose → G6P (Hexo/Glucokinase)
  - F6P → F 1,6 BP (PFK1)
  - PEP → pyruvate (pyruvate kinase)

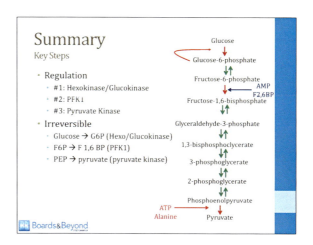

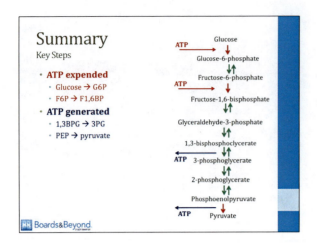

Gluconeogenesis

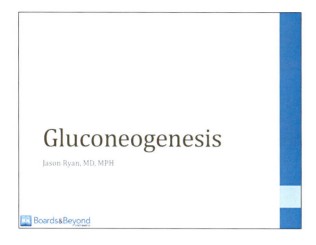
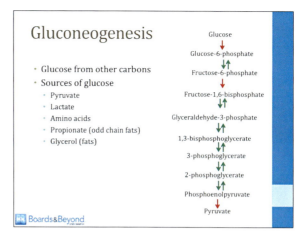
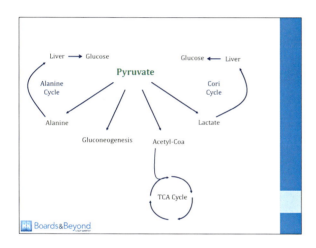
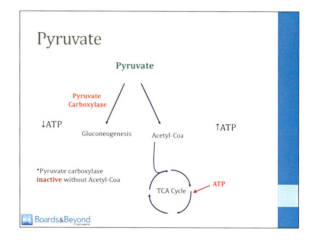
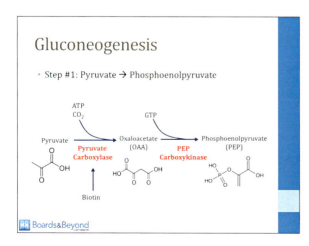
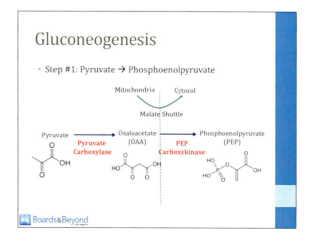

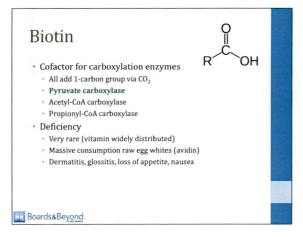

Biotin

- Cofactor for carboxylation enzymes
  - All add 1-carbon group via CO_2
  - **Pyruvate carboxylase**
  - Acetyl-CoA carboxylase
  - Propionyl-CoA carboxylase
- Deficiency
  - Very rare (vitamin widely distributed)
  - Massive consumption raw egg whites (avidin)
  - Dermatitis, glossitis, loss of appetite, nausea

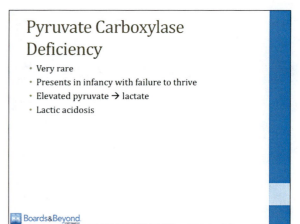

Pyruvate Carboxylase Deficiency

- Very rare
- Presents in infancy with failure to thrive
- Elevated pyruvate → lactate
- Lactic acidosis

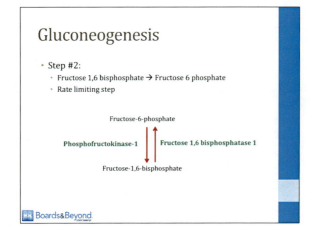

Gluconeogenesis

- Step #2:
  - Fructose 1,6 bisphosphate → Fructose 6 phosphate
  - Rate limiting step

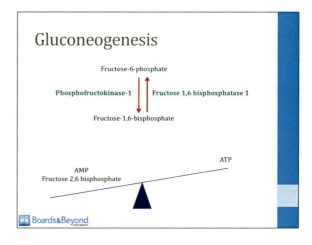

Gluconeogenesis

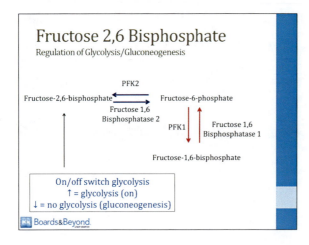

Fructose 2,6 Bisphosphate
Regulation of Glycolysis/Gluconeogenesis

On/off switch glycolysis
↑ = glycolysis (on)
↓ = no glycolysis (gluconeogenesis)

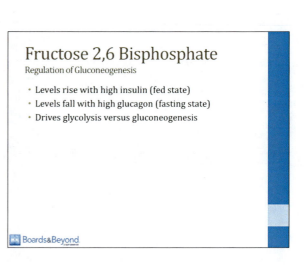

Fructose 2,6 Bisphosphate
Regulation of Gluconeogenesis

- Levels rise with high insulin (fed state)
- Levels fall with high glucagon (fasting state)
- Drives glycolysis versus gluconeogenesis

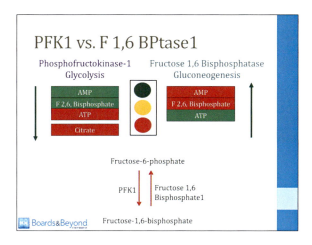

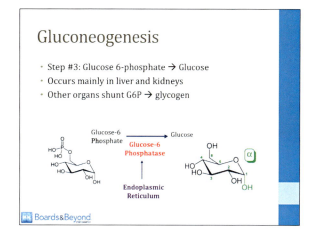

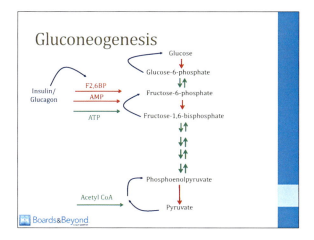

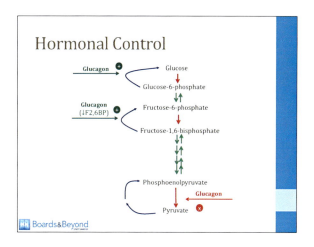

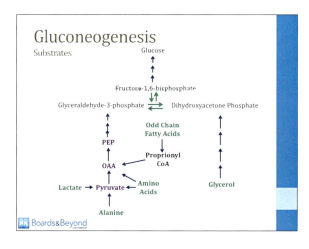

Hormones

- Insulin
  - Shuts down gluconeogenesis (favors glycolysis)
  - Action via F 2,6, BP
- Glucagon (opposite of insulin)

Other Hormones

- Epinephrine
  - Raises blood glucose
  - Gluconeogenesis and glycogen breakdown
- Cortisol
  - Increases gluconeogenesis enzymes
  - **Hyperglycemia** common side effect steroid drugs
- Thyroid hormone
  - Increases gluconeogenesis

Glycogen

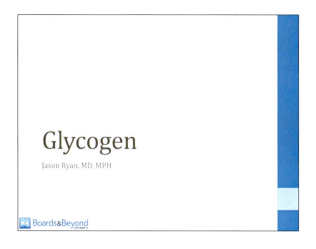
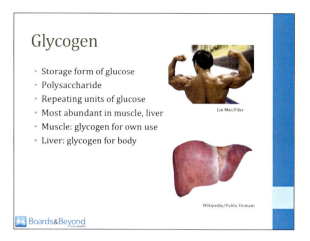
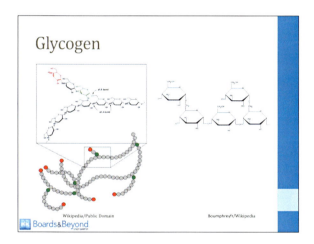
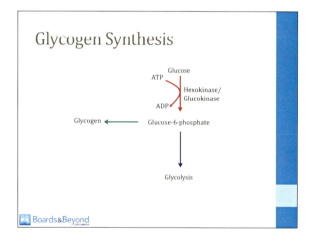
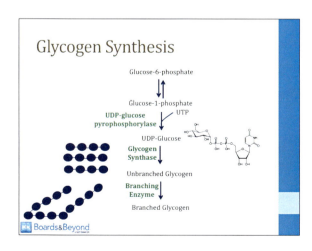
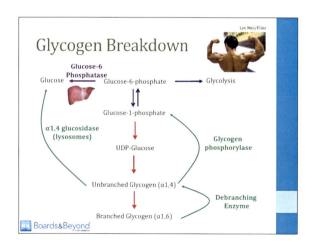

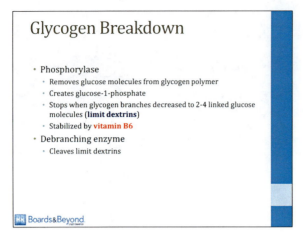
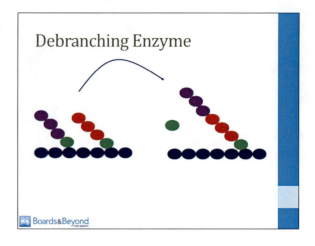
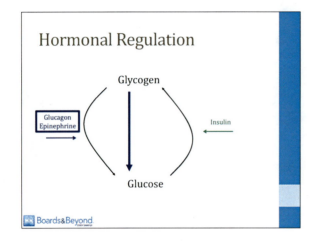
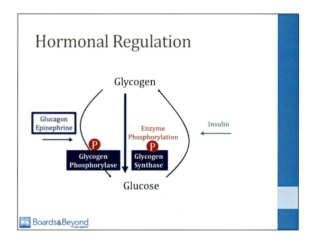
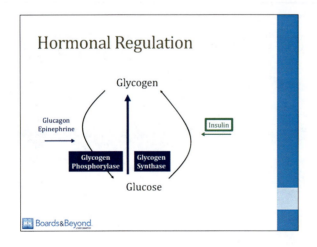
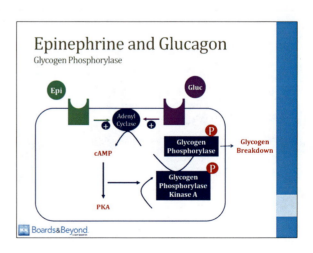

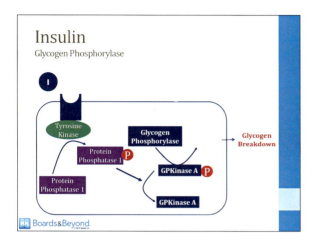
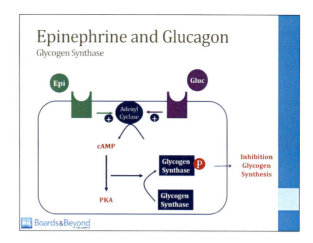
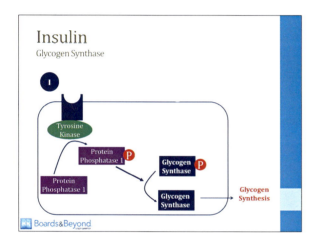
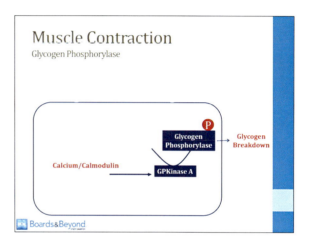
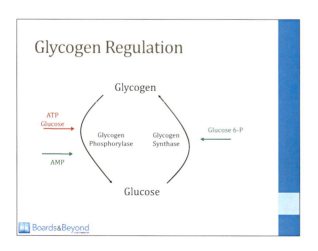
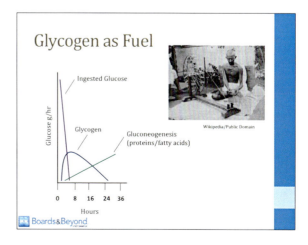

Glycogen Storage Diseases

- Most autosomal recessive
- Defective breakdown of glycogen
- Liver: hypoglycemia
- Muscle: weakness
- More than 14 described

Von Gierke's Disease
Glycogen Storage Disease Type I

- Glucose-6-phosphatase deficiency (Type Ia)
  - Type Ib: Glucose transporter deficiency
- Presents in infancy: 2-6 months of age
- Severe hypoglycemia between meals
  - Lethargy
  - Seizures
  - Lactic acidosis (Cori cycle)
- Enlarged liver (excess glycogen)
  - Can lead to liver failure

Cori Cycle
Lactate Cycle

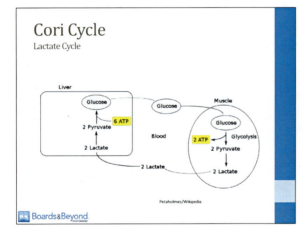

Von Gierke's Disease
Glycogen Storage Disease Type I

- Diagnosis:
  - DNA testing (preferred)
  - Liver biopsy (historical test)
- Treatment: Cornstarch (glucose polymer)
- Avoid sucrose, lactose, fructose, galactose
  - Feed into glycolysis pathways
  - Cannot be metabolized to glucose via gluconeogenesis
  - Worsen accumulation of glucose 6-phosphate

Pompe's Disease
Glycogen Storage Disease Type II

- Acid alpha-glucosidase deficiency
  - Also "lysosomal acid maltase"
- Accumulation of glycogen in lysosomes
- Classic form presents in infancy
- Severe disease → often death in infancy/childhood

Pompe's Disease
Glycogen Storage Disease Type II

- Enlarged muscles
  - Cardiomegaly
  - Enlarged tongue
- Hypotonia
- Liver enlargement (often from heart failure)
- No metabolic problems (hypoglycemia)
- Death from heart failure

Cori's Disease
Glycogen Storage Disease Type III

- Debranching enzyme deficiency
- Similar to type I except:
  - Milder hypoglycemia
  - No lactic acidosis (Cori cycle intact)
  - Muscle involvement (glycogen accumulation)
- Key point: Gluconeogenesis is **intact**

Cori's Disease
Glycogen Storage Disease Type III

- Classic presentation:
  - Infant or child with hypoglycemia/hepatomegaly
  - Hypotonia/weakness
  - Possible cardiomyopathy with hypertrophy

McArdle's Disease
Glycogen Storage Disease Type V

- Muscle glycogen phosphorylase deficiency
  - Myophosphorylase deficiency
  - Skeletal muscle has unique isoform of G-phosphorylase
- Glycogen not properly broken down in muscle cells
- Usually presents in **adolescence/early adulthood**
  - Exercise intolerance, fatigue, **cramps**
  - Poor endurance, muscle swelling, and weakness
  - **Myoglobinuria** and CK release (especially with exercise)
  - Urine may turn dark after exercise

Glycogen Synthase Deficiency

- Can't form liver glycogen normally
- **Fasting hypoglycemia** with ketosis
- Postprandial hyperglycemia
- May present in older children (less frequent feeds)
- **Morning fatigue**
- Symptoms improve with food

HMP Shunt

HMP Shunt
Jason Ryan, MD, MPH

HMP Shunt
- Series of reactions that goes by several names:
  - Hexose monophosphate shunt
  - Pentose phosphate pathway
  - 6-phosphogluconate pathway
- Glucose 6-phosphate "shunted" away from glycolysis

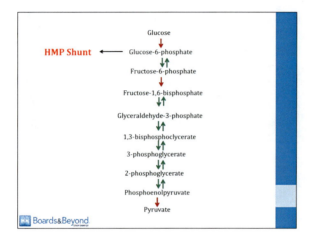

HMP Shunt
- Synthesizes:
  - **NADPH** (many uses)
  - **Ribose 5-phosphate** (nucleotide synthesis)
- Two key clinical correlations:
  - **G6PD deficiency**
  - **Thiamine deficiency (transketolase)**

HMP Shunt
- All reactions occur in cytosol
- Two phases:
  - Oxidative: irreversible, rate-limiting
  - Reductive: reversible

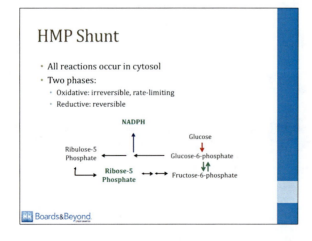

HMP Shunt
Oxidative Reactions

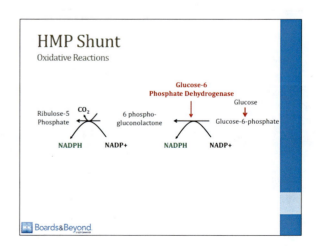

HMP Shunt
Reductive Reactions

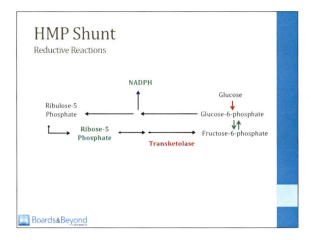

Transketolase

- Transfers a carbon unit to create F-6-phosphate
- Requires **thiamine (B1)** as a co-factor
- **Wernicke-Korsakoff syndrome**
  - Abnormal transketolase may predispose
  - Affected individuals may have abnormal binding to thiamine

Ribose-5-Phosphate

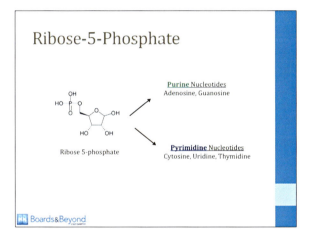

NADPH
Nicotinamide adenine dinucleotide phosphate

- Similar structure to NADH
- Not used for oxidative phosphorylation (ATP)

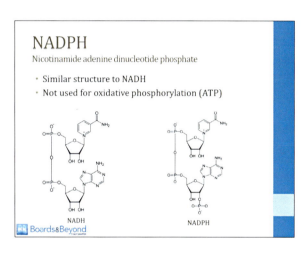

NADPH Uses

- Used in "reductive" reactions
- Releases hydrogen to form NADP⁺
- Use #1: Co-factor in **fatty acid, steroid synthesis**
  - Liver, mammary glands, testis, adrenal cortex
- Use #2: **Phagocytosis**
- Use #3: Protection from **oxidative damage**

Respiratory Burst

- Phagocytes generate H_2O_2 to kill bacteria
  - "Oxygen dependent" killing
  - "Oxygen independent": low pH, enzymes
- Uses three key enzymes:
  - NADPH oxidase
  - Superoxide dismutase
  - Myeloperoxidase

Respiratory Burst

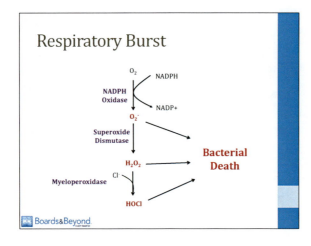

CGD
Chronic Granulomatous Disease

- Loss of function of NADPH oxidase
- Phagocytes cannot generate H_2O_2
- Catalase (-) bacteria generate their own H_2O_2
  - Phagocytes use despite enzyme deficiency
- **Catalase (+) bacteria** breakdown H_2O_2
  - Host cells have no H_2O_2 to use → recurrent infections
- Five organisms cause almost all CGD infections:
  - Staph aureus, Pseudomonas, Serratia, Nocardia, Aspergillus

Source: UpToDate

G6PD Deficiency
Glucose-6-Phosphate Dehydrogenase

- NADPH required for normal red blood cell function
- H_2O_2 generation triggered in RBCs
  - Infections
  - Drugs
  - Fava beans
- Need NADPH to degrade H_2O_2
- Absence of required NADPH → hemolysis

Glutathione
Erythrocytes

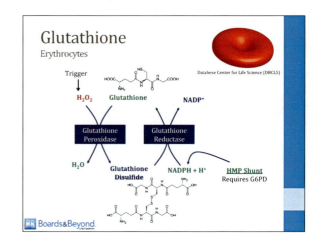

G6PD Deficiency
Glucose-6-Phosphate Dehydrogenase

- **X-linked** disorder (males)
- Most common human enzyme disorder
- High prevalence in **Africa**, Asia, the Mediterranean
  - May protect against malaria
- **Recurrent hemolysis** after exposure to trigger
  May present as dark urine
- Other HMP functions usually okay
  - Nucleic acids, fatty acids, etc.

G6PD Deficiency
Glucose-6-Phosphate Dehydrogenase

- Classic findings: **Heinz bodies** and **bite cells**
- Heinz bodies: oxidized Hgb precipitated in RBCs
- Bite cells: phagocytic removal by splenic macrophages

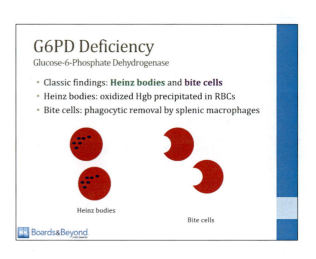

Heinz bodies — Bite cells

G6PD Deficiency
Triggers

- Infection: Macrophages generate free radicals
- Fava beans: Contain oxidants
- Drugs:
  - Antibiotics (**sulfa drugs**, dapsone, nitrofurantoin, INH)
  - **Anti-malarials** (primaquine, quinidine)
  - Aspirin, acetaminophen (rare)

G6PD Deficiency
Diagnosis and Treatment

- Diagnosis:
  - Fluorescent spot test
  - Detects generation of NADPH from NADP
  - Positive test if blood spot fails to fluoresce under UV light
- Treatment:
  - Avoidance of triggers

Fructose and Galactose

Fructose and Galactose
Jason Ryan, MD, MPH

Fructose and Galactose
- Isomers of glucose (same formula: $C_6H_{12}O_6$)
- Galactose (and glucose) taken up by SGLT1
  - Na+ dependent transporter
- Fructose taken up by facilitated diffusion GLUT-5
- All leave enterocytes by GLUT-2

Carbohydrate GI Absorption
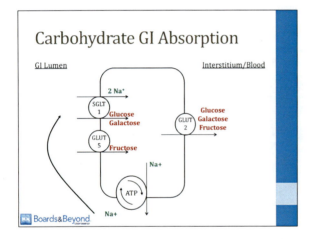

Fructose
- Commonly found in **sucrose** (glucose + fructose)
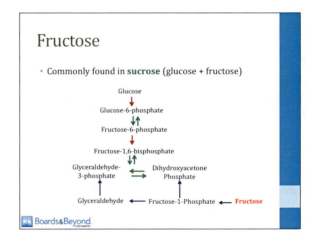

Fructose
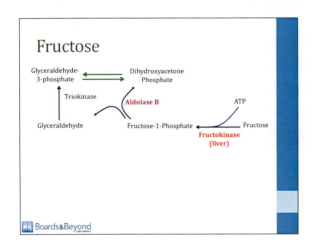

Fructose
Special Point

Phosphofructokinase-1
Rate-limiting step: glycolysis

Fructose bypasses PFK-1
Rapid metabolism

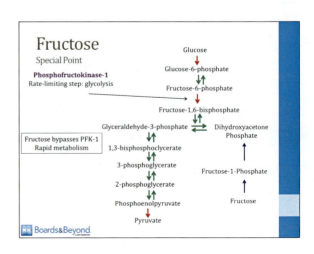

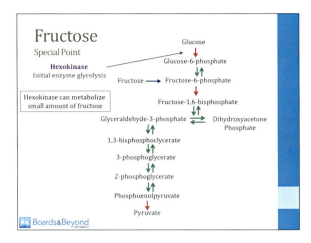

Essential Fructosuria

- Deficiency of **fructokinase**
- Benign condition
- Fructose not taken up by liver cells
- Fructose appears in urine (depending on intake)

Hereditary Fructose Intolerance

- Deficiency of **aldolase B**
- Build-up of fructose 1-phosphate
- Depletion of ATP

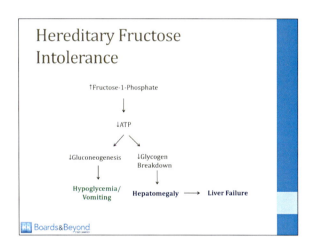

Hereditary Fructose Intolerance

- Baby **just weaned from breast milk**
- Failure to thrive
- Symptoms after feeding
  - **Hypoglycemia (seizures)**
- Enlarged liver
- Part of newborn screening panel
- Treatment:
  - Avoid fructose, sucrose, sorbitol

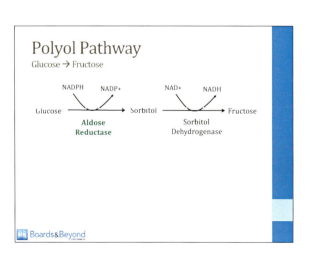

Galactose

- Commonly found in **lactose** (glucose + galactose)
- Converted to glucose 6-phosphate

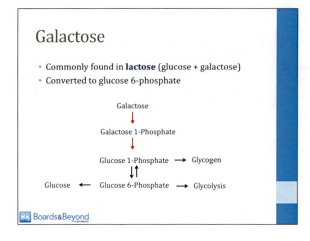

Galactose

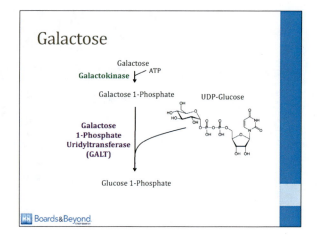

Classic Galactosemia

- Deficiency of galactose 1-phosphate uridyltransferase
- Autosomal recessive disorder
- Galactose-1-phosphate accumulates in cells
- Leads to accumulation of galactitol in cells

Polyol Pathway

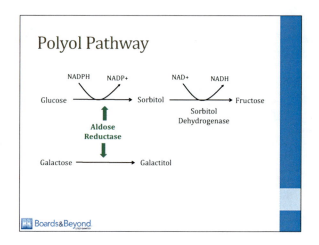

Classic Galactosemia

- Presents in infancy
  - Often first few days of life
  - Shortly after consumption of milk
- Liver accumulation galactose/galactitol
  - Liver failure
  - Jaundice
  - Hepatomegaly
  - Failure to thrive
- Cataracts if untreated

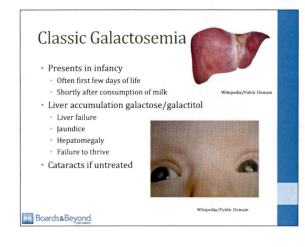

Classic Galactosemia

- Screening: GALT enzyme activity assay
- Treatment: avoid galactose

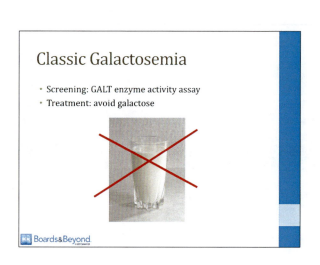

Galactokinase Deficiency

- Milder form of galactosemia
- Galactose not taken up by cells
- Accumulates in **blood** and **urine**
- Main problem: **cataracts** as child/young adult
    - May present as vision problems

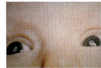

Pyruvate Dehydrogenase

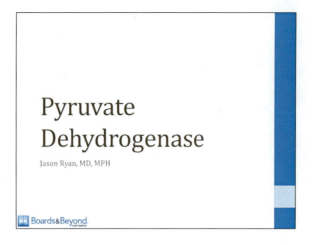
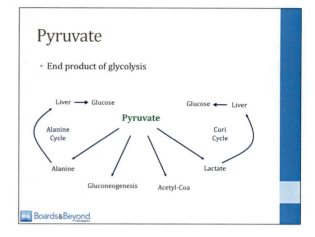
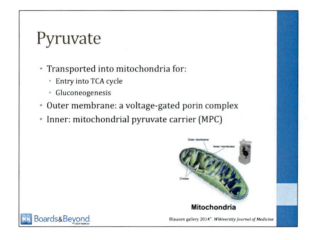
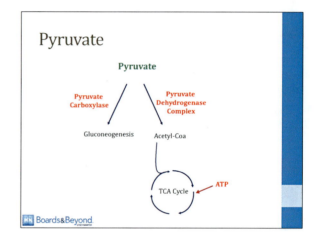
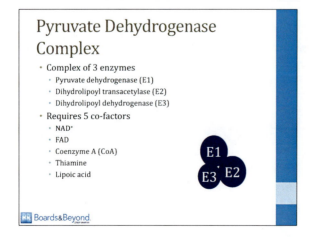
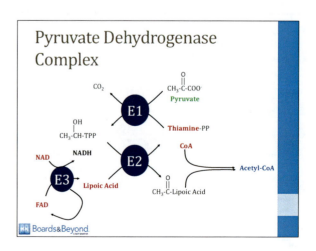

Thiamine
PDH Cofactors

- **Vitamin B1**
- Converted to thiamine pyrophosphate (TPP)
- Co-factor for **four** enzymes
  - Pyruvate dehydrogenase
  - α-ketoglutarate dehydrogenase (TCA cycle)
  - α-ketoacid dehydrogenase (branched chain amino acids)
  - Transketolase (HMP shunt)

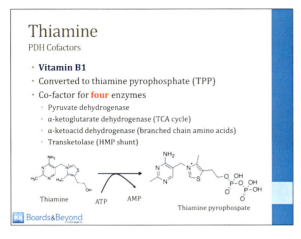

Thiamine Deficiency

- ↓ production of ATP
- ↑ aerobic tissues affected most (nerves/heart)
- **Beriberi**
  - Underdeveloped areas
  - Dry type: polyneuritis, muscle weakness
  - Wet type: tachycardia, high-output heart failure, edema
- **Wernicke-Korsakoff syndrome**
  - Alcoholics (malnourished, poor absorption vitamins)
  - Confusion, confabulation

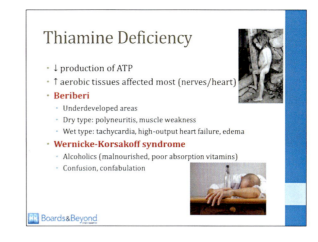

Thiamine and Glucose

- Malnourished patients: ↓glucose ↓thiamine
- If glucose given first → unable to metabolize
- Case reports of worsening Wernicke-Korsakoff

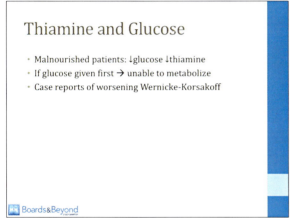

FAD
PDH Cofactors

- Synthesized from **riboflavin (B2)**
- Added to adenosine → FAD
- Accepts 2 electrons → FADH2

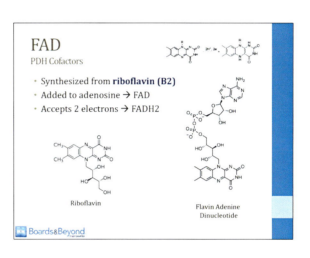

NAD$^+$
PDH Cofactors

- Carries electrons as NADH
- Synthesized from **niacin (B3)**
  - Niacin: synthesized from tryptophan
- Used in electron transport

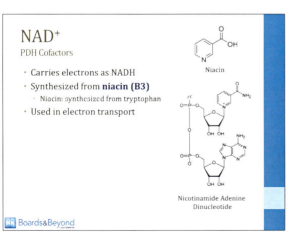

Coenzyme A
PDH Cofactors

- Also a nucleotide coenzyme (NAD, FAD)
- Synthesized from **pantothenic acid (B5)**
- Accepts/donates acyl groups

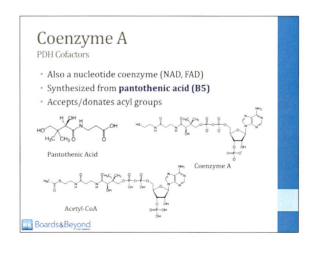

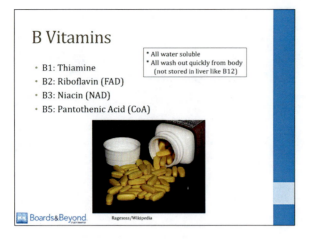

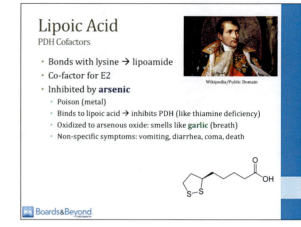

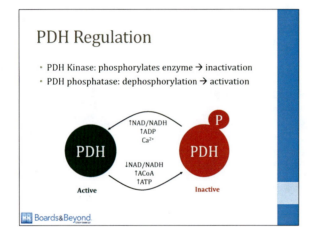

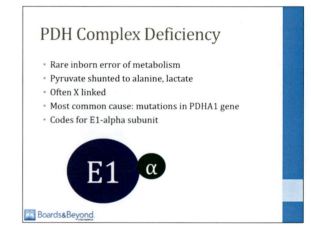

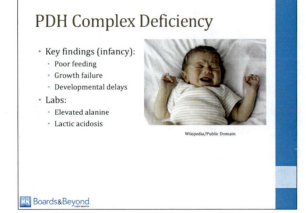

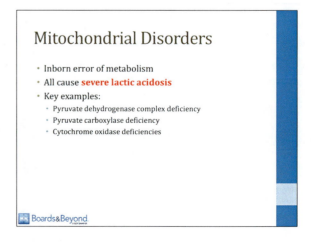

PDH Complex Deficiency
Treatment

- Thiamine, lipoic acid (optimize remaining PDH)
- Ketogenic diet
  - Low carbohydrates (reduces lactic acidosis)
  - High fat
  - Ketogenic amino acids: Lysine and leucine
  - Drives ketone production (instead of glucose)

Ketogenic Amino Acids

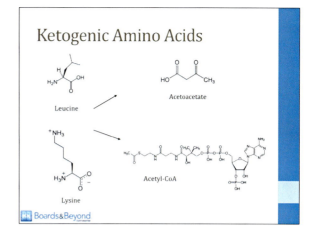

TCA Cycle

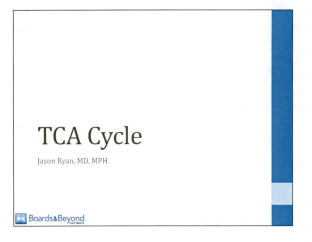

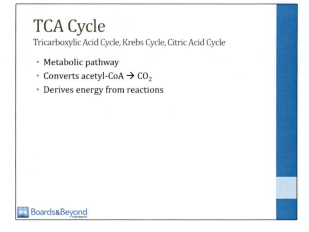

TCA Cycle
Tricarboxylic Acid Cycle, Krebs Cycle, Citric Acid Cycle

- Metabolic pathway
- Converts acetyl-CoA → CO_2
- Derives energy from reactions

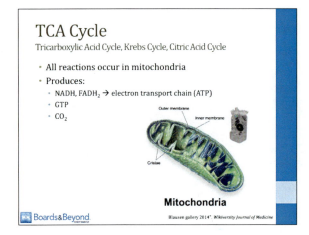

TCA Cycle
Tricarboxylic Acid Cycle, Krebs Cycle, Citric Acid Cycle

- All reactions occur in mitochondria
- Produces:
  - NADH, $FADH_2$ → electron transport chain (ATP)
  - GTP
  - CO_2

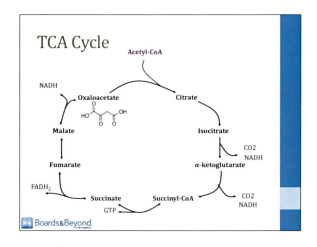

TCA Cycle

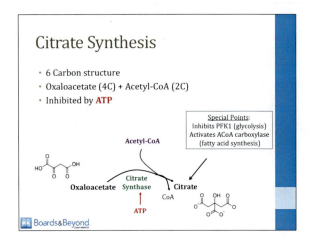

Citrate Synthesis

- 6 Carbon structure
- Oxaloacetate (4C) + Acetyl-CoA (2C)
- Inhibited by **ATP**

Special Points:
Inhibits PFK1 (glycolysis)
Activates ACoA carboxylase
(fatty acid synthesis)

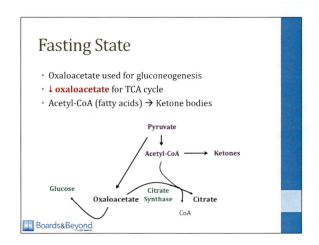

Fasting State

- Oxaloacetate used for gluconeogenesis
- ↓ **oxaloacetate** for TCA cycle
- Acetyl-CoA (fatty acids) → Ketone bodies

Isocitrate

- Isomer of citrate
- Enzyme: aconitase
- Forms intermediate (cis-aconitate) then isocitrate
- Inhibited by fluoroacetate: rat poison

α-Ketoglutarate

- Rate limiting step of TCA cycle
- Inhibited by:
  - ATP
  - NADH
- Activated by:
  - ADP
  - Ca++

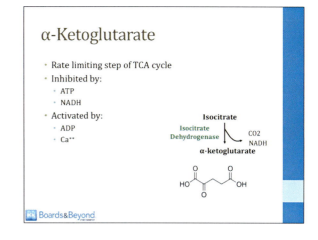

Succinyl-CoA

- α-ketoglutarate dehydrogenase complex
- Similar to pyruvate dehydrogenase complex
- Cofactors:
  - Thiamine
  - CoA
  - NAD
  - FADH
  - Lipoic acid

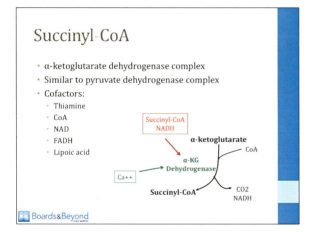

Succinate

- Succinyl-CoA synthetase

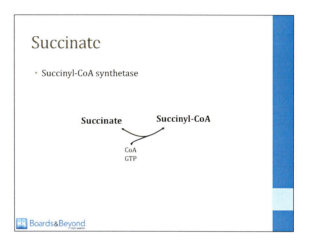

Fumarate

- Succinate dehydrogenase
- Unique enzyme: embedded mitochondrial membrane
- Functions as complex II electron transport

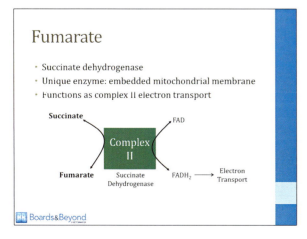

Fumarate

- Also produced several other pathways
  - Urea cycle
  - Purine synthesis (formation of IMP)
  - Amino acid breakdown: phenylalanine, tyrosine

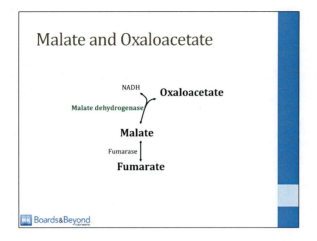
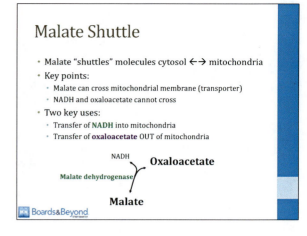
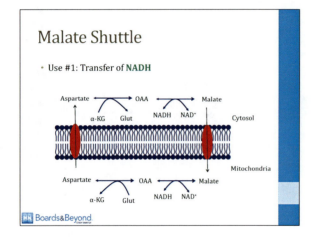
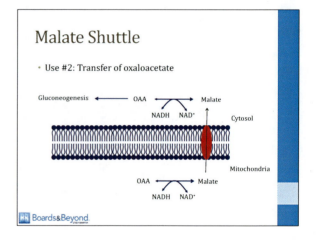
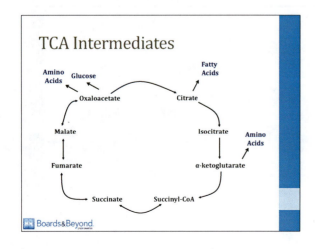
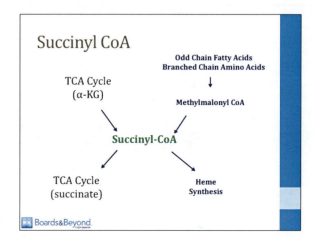

TCA Cycle
Key Points

- Inhibited by:
  - ATP
  - NADH
  - Acetyl CoA
  - Citrate
  - Succinyl CoA

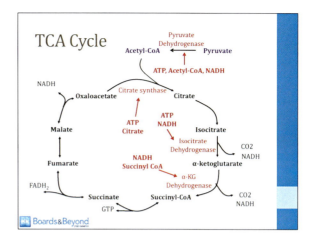

TCA Cycle
Key Points

- Activated by:
  - ADP
  - Calcium

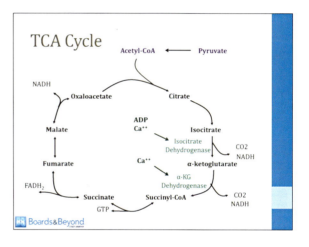

Electron Transport Chain

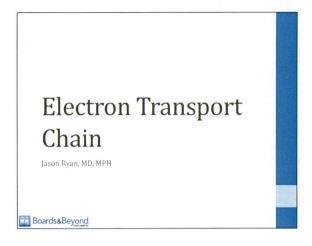

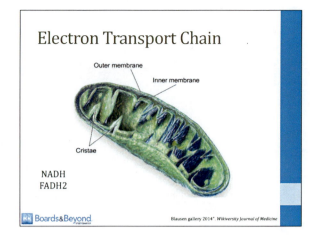

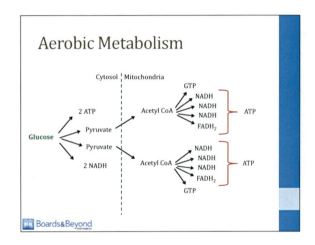

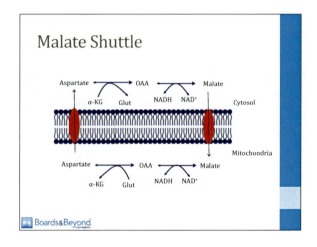

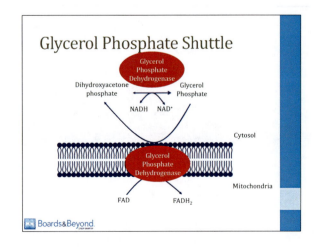

Electron Transport

- Extract electrons from NADH/FADH$_2$
- Transfer to **oxygen** (*aerobic* respiration)
- In process, generate/capture energy
- NADH → NAD$^+$ + H$^+$ + 2e$^-$
- FADH$_2$ → FAD$^+$ + 2 H$^+$ + 2e$^-$
- 2e$^-$ + 2H$^+$ + ½O$_2$ → H$_2$O

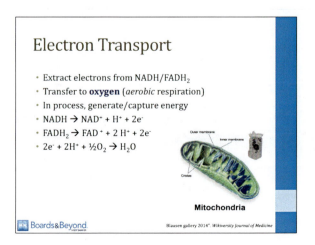

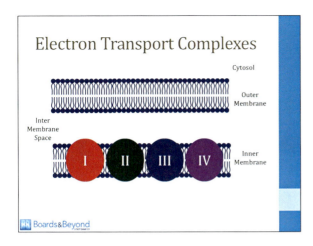

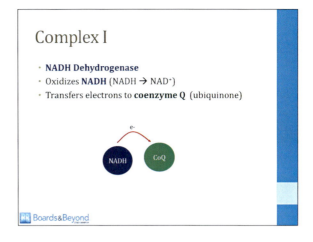

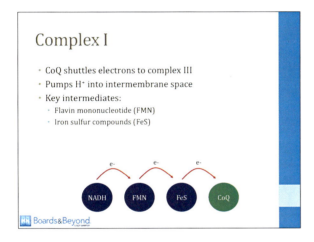

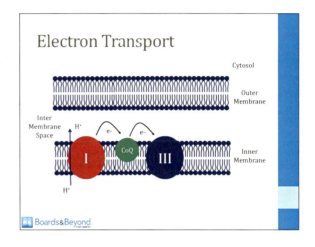

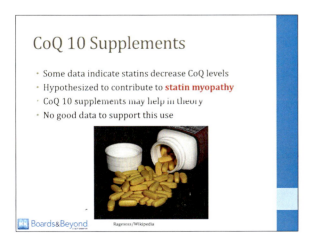

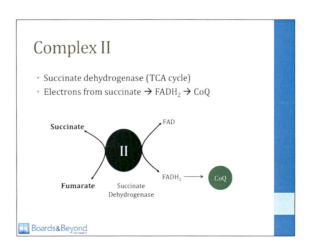

Complex III

- **Cytochrome bc_1** complex
- Transfers electrons CoQ → **cytochrome c**
- Pumps H^+ to intermembrane space

Electron Transport

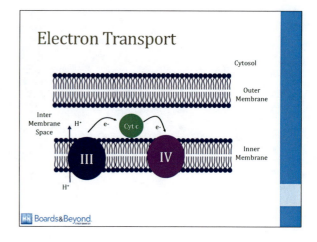

Cytochromes

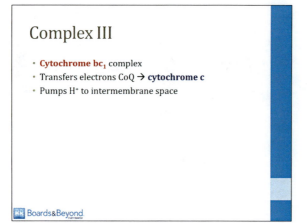

- Class of **proteins**
- Contains a **heme** group
- Iron plus **porphyrin** ring
- Hgb: **mostly Fe^{2+}**
- Cytochromes: $Fe^{2+} \leftrightarrow Fe^{3+}$
- Oxidation state changes with electron transport
- Electron transport: a, b, c
- Cytochrome P450: drug metabolism

Complex IV

- Cytochrome **a + a3**
- **Cytochrome c oxidase** (reacts with oxygen)
- Contains **copper (Cu)**
- Electrons and O_2 → H_2O
- Also pumps H^+

Electron Transport

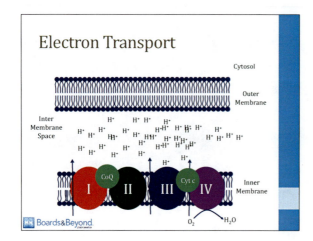

Phosphorylation

- Two ways to produce ATP:
  - Substrate level phosphorylation
  - Oxidative phosphorylation
- Substrate level phosphorylation (via enzyme):

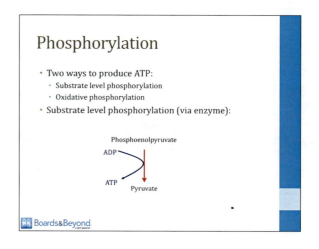

Oxidative Phosphorylation

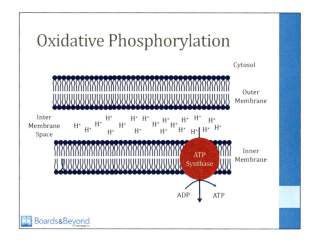

ATP Synthase

- **Complex V**
- Converts proton (charge) gradient → ATP
  - "electrochemical gradient"
  - "proton motive force"
- Protons move down gradient ("chemiosmosis")

P/O Ratio

- ATP per molecule O_2
- Classically had to be an integer
  - 3 per NADH
  - 2 per $FADH_2$
- Newer estimates
  - 2.5 per NADH
  - 1.5 per $FADH_2$

Hinkle P. P/O ratios of mitochondrial oxidative phosphorylation. Biochimica et Biophysica Act 1706 (Jan 2005) 1-11

Aerobic Energy Production

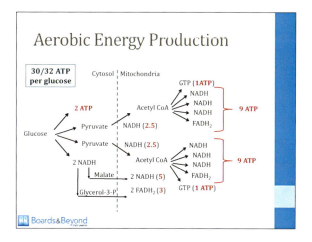

Drugs and Poisons

- Two ways to disrupt oxidative phosphorylation
- #1: Block/inhibit electron transport
- #2: Allow H^+ to leak out of inner membrane space
  - "**Uncoupling**" of electron transport/oxidative phosphorylation

Inhibitors

- Rotenone (insecticide)
  - Binds complex I
  - Prevents electron transfer (reduction) to CoQ
- Antimycin A (antibiotic)
  - Complex III (bc1 complex)
- Complex IV
  - Carbon monoxide (binds a3 in Fe^{2+} state – competes with O_2)
  - Cyanide (binds a3 in Fe^{3+} state)

Cyanide Poisoning

- CNS: Headache, confusion
- Cardiovascular: Initial tachycardia, hypertension
- Respiratory: Initial tachypnea
- **Bright red** venous blood: ↑O_2 content
- Almond smell
- Anaerobic metabolism: **lactic acidosis**

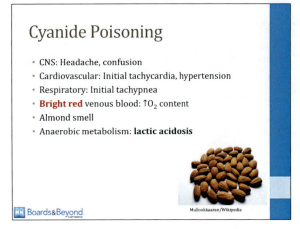

Cyanide Poisoning

- **Nitroprusside**: treatment of hypertensive emergencies
  - Contains five cyanide groups per molecule
  - Toxic levels with prolonged infusions
- Treatment: **Nitrites** (amyl nitrite)
  - Converts Fe^{2+} → Fe^{3+} in Hgb (methemoglobin)
  - Fe^{3+} in Hgb binds cyanide, protects mitochondria

Uncoupling Agents

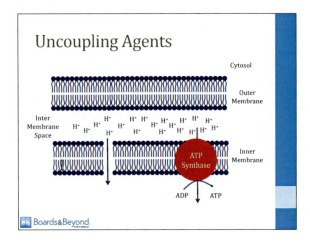

Uncoupling Agents

- 2,4 dinitrophenol (DNP)
- **Aspirin (overdose)**
- **Brown fat**
  - Newborns (also hibernating animals)
  - **Uncoupling protein 1 (UCP-1, thermogenin)**
  - Sympathetic stimulation (NE, β receptors) → lipolysis
  - Electron transport → heat (not ATP)

All lead to production of *heat*

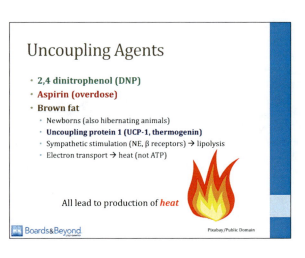

Oligomycin A

- Macrolide antibiotic
- **Inhibits ATP synthase**
- Protons cannot move through enzyme
- Protons trapped in intermembrane space
- Oxidative phosphorylation stops
- ATP cannot be generated

Fatty Acids

Fatty Acids

Jason Ryan, MD, MPH

Lipids

- Mostly carbon and hydrogen
- Not soluble in water
- Many types:
  - Fatty acids
  - Triacylglycerol (triglycerides)
  - Cholesterol
  - Phospholipids
  - Steroids
  - Glycolipids

Lipids

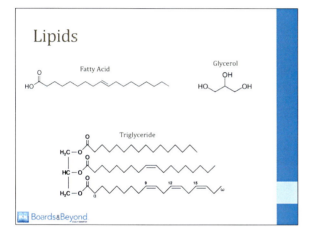

Fatty Acid and Triglycerides

- Most lipids degraded to **free fatty acids** in intestine
- Enterocytes convert FAs to **triacylglycerol**
- **Chylomicrons** carry through plasma
- TAG degraded back to free fatty acids
  - **Lipoprotein lipase**
  - Endothelial surfaces of capillaries
  - Abundant in adipocytes and muscle tissue

Vocabulary

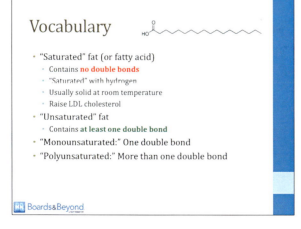

- "Saturated" fat (or fatty acid)
  - Contains **no double bonds**
  - "Saturated" with hydrogen
  - Usually solid at room temperature
  - Raise LDL cholesterol
- "Unsaturated" fat
  - Contains **at least one double bond**
- "Monounsaturated:" One double bond
- "Polyunsaturated:" More than one double bond

More Vocabulary

- Trans fat
  - Double bonds (unsaturated) can be trans or cis
  - Most natural fats have cis configuration
  - Trans from partial hydrogenation (food processing method)
  - Can increase LDL, lower HDL
- Omega-3 fatty acids
  - Type of polyunsaturated fat
  - Found in fish oil
  - Lower triglyceride levels

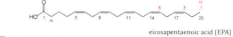

eicosapentaenoic acid (EPA)

Fatty Acid Metabolism

- Fatty acids **synthesis**
  - Liver, mammary glands, adipose tissue (small amount)
  - Excess carbohydrates and proteins → fatty acids
- Fatty acid **storage**
  - Adipose tissue
  - Stored as triglycerides
- Fatty acid breakdown
  - **β-oxidation**
  - Acetyl CoA → TCA cycle → ATP

Fatty Acid Synthesis

- In high energy states (fed state):
  - Lots of acetyl-CoA
  - Lots of ATP
  - Inhibition of isocitrate dehydrogenase (TCA cycle)
- Result: **High citrate level**

Fatty Acid Synthesis

- Step 1: Citrate to cytosol via citrate shuttle
- Key point: Acetyl-CoA cannot cross membrane

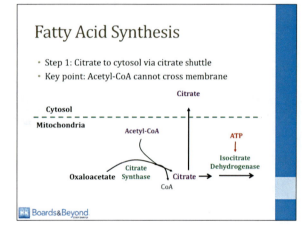

Fatty Acid Synthesis

- Step 2: Citrate converted to acetyl-CoA
- Net effect: Excess acetyl-CoA moved to cytosol

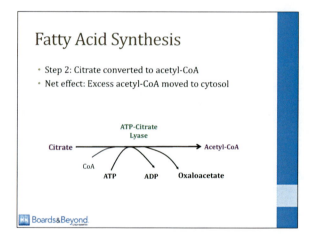

Fatty Acid Synthesis

- Step 3: Acetyl-CoA converted to malonyl-CoA
- Rate limiting step

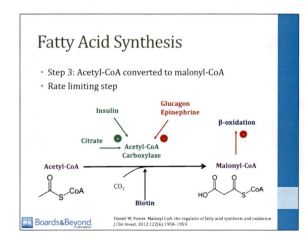

Daniel W. Foster. Malonyl CoA: the regulator of fatty acid synthesis and oxidation
J Clin Invest. 2012;122(6):1958-1959.

Biotin

- Cofactor for carboxylation enzymes
  - All **add 1-carbon group** via CO_2
  - Pyruvate carboxylase
  - **Acetyl-CoA carboxylase**
  - Propionyl-CoA carboxylase

Fatty Acid Synthesis

- Step #4: Synthesis of palmitate
- Enzyme: **fatty acid synthase**
- Uses carbons from acetyl CoA and malonyl CoA
- Creates **16 carbon** fatty acid
- Requires **NADPH** (HMP Shunt)

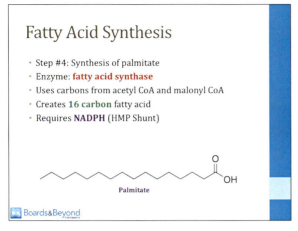
Palmitate

Fatty Acid Storage

- Palmitate can be modified to other fatty acids
- Used by various tissues based on needs
- Stored as triacylglycerols in adipose tissue

Fatty Acid Breakdown

- Key enzyme: **Hormone sensitive lipase**
- Removes fatty acids from TAG in adipocytes
- Activated by **glucagon** and **epinephrine**

Fatty Acid Breakdown

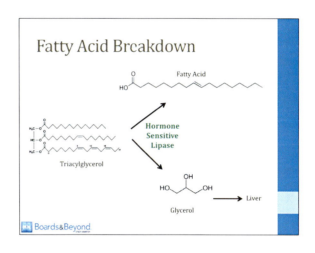

Glycerol

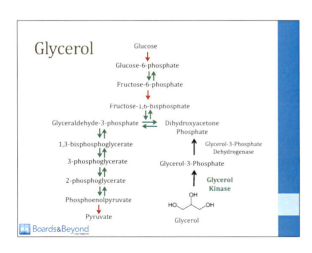

Fatty Acid Breakdown

- Fatty acids transported via **albumin**
- Taken up by tissues
- Not used by:
  - **RBCs**: Glycolysis only (no mitochondria)
  - **Brain**: Glucose and ketones only

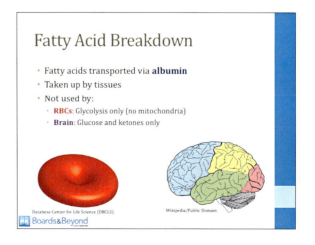

Fatty Acid Breakdown

- **β-oxidation**
- Removal of 2-carbon units from fatty acids
- Produces acetyl-CoA, NADH, FADH$_2$

β-oxidation

- Step #1: Convert fatty acid to fatty acyl CoA

β-oxidation

- Step #2: Transport fatty acyl CoA → inner mitochondria
- Uses **carnitine shuttle**
- Carnitine in diet
- Also synthesized from lysine and methionine
  - **Only liver, kidney** can synthesize de novo
  - **Muscle and heart** depend on diet or other tissues

Carnitine

Carnitine Shuttle

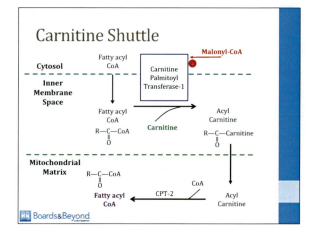

Carnitine Deficiencies

- Several potential secondary causes
  - Malnutrition
  - Liver disease
  - Increased requirements (trauma, burns, pregnancy)
  - Hemodialysis (↓ synthesis; loss through membranes)
- Major consequence:
  - Inability to transport LCFA to mitochondria
  - Accumulation of LCFA in cells
- Low serum **carnitine** and **acylcarnitine** levels

Carnitine Deficiencies

- **Muscle** weakness, especially during exercise
- **Cardiomyopathy**
- **Hypoketotic hypoglycemia** when fasting
  - Tissues overuse glucose
  - Poor ketone synthesis without fatty acid breakdown

Primary systemic carnitine deficiency

- Mutation affecting carnitine **uptake** into cells
- Infantile phenotype presents first two year of life
  - Encephalopathy
  - Hepatomegaly
  - Hyperammonemia (liver dysfunction)
  - Hypoketotic hypoglycemia
  - Low serum carnitine: kidneys cannot resorb carnitine
  - Reduced carnitine levels in muscle, liver, and heart

β-oxidation

- Step #3: Begin "cycles" of beta oxidation
- Removes two carbons
- Shortens chain by two
- Generates NADH, FADH2, Acetyl CoA

β-oxidation

- First step in a cycle involves **acyl-CoA dehydrogenase**
- Adds a double bond between α and β carbons

Acyl-CoA Dehydrogenase

- Family of four enzymes
  - Short
  - Medium
  - Long
  - Very-long chain fatty acids
- Well described deficiency of medium chain enzyme

MCAD Deficiency
Medium Chain Acyl-CoA Dehydrogenase

- Autosomal recessive disorder
- Poor oxidation 6-10 carbon fatty acids
- Severe **hypoglycemia without ketones**
- Dicarboxylic acids 6-10 carbons in urine
- **High acylcarnitine levels**

Dicarboxylic Acid

MCAD Deficiency
Medium Chain Acyl-CoA Dehydrogenase

- **Gluconeogenesis shutdown**
  - Pyruvate carboxylase depends on Acetyl-CoA
  - Acetyl-CoA levels low in absence β-oxidation
- Exacerbated in **fasting/infection**
- Treatment: Avoid fasting

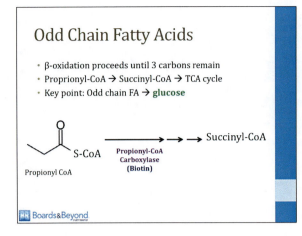
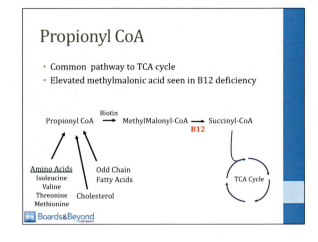

Methylmalonic Acidemia

- Deficiency of **Methylmalonyl-CoA mutase**
- Anion gap metabolic acidosis
- CNS dysfunction
- Often fatal early in life

Ketone Bodies

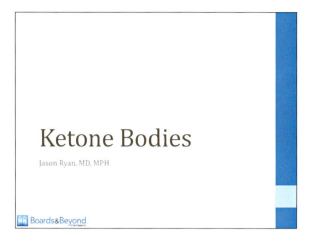

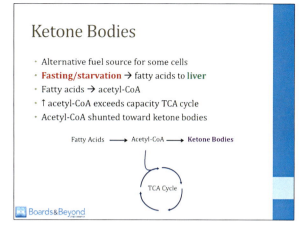

Ketone Bodies

- Alternative fuel source for some cells
- **Fasting/starvation** → fatty acids to **liver**
- Fatty acids → acetyl-CoA
- ↑ acetyl-CoA exceeds capacity TCA cycle
- Acetyl-CoA shunted toward ketone bodies

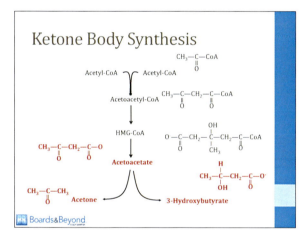

Ketone Body Synthesis

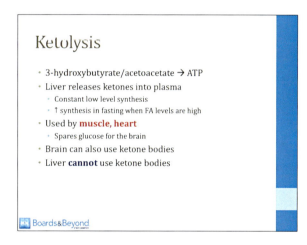

Ketolysis

- 3-hydroxybutyrate/acetoacetate → ATP
- Liver releases ketones into plasma
  - Constant low level synthesis
  - ↑ synthesis in fasting when FA levels are high
- Used by **muscle, heart**
  - Spares glucose for the brain
- Brain can also use ketone bodies
- Liver **cannot** use ketone bodies

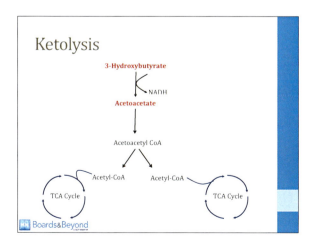

Ketolysis

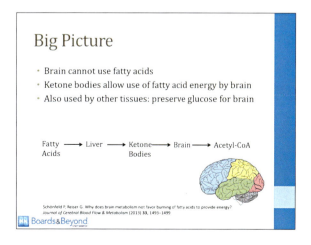

Big Picture

- Brain cannot use fatty acids
- Ketone bodies allow use of fatty acid energy by brain
- Also used by other tissues: preserve glucose for brain

Schönfeld P, Reiser G. Why does brain metabolism not favor burning of fatty acids to provide energy? *Journal of Cerebral Blood Flow & Metabolism* (2013) 33, 1493–1499

Ketoacidosis

- Ketone bodies have low pKa
- Release H^+ at plasma pH
- ↑ ketones → anion gap metabolic acidosis

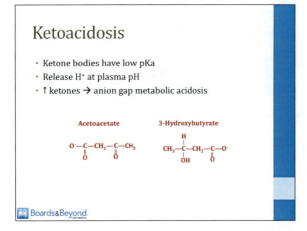

Diabetes

- Low insulin
- High fatty acid utilization
- Oxaloacetate depleted
- TCA cycle stalls
- ↑ acetyl-CoA
- Ketone production

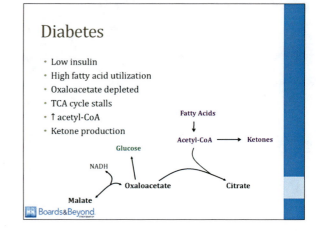

Alcoholism

- EtOH metabolism: excess NADH
- Oxaloacetate shunted to malate
- Stalls TCA cycle
- ↑ acetyl-CoA
- Ketone production
- Also ↓ gluconeogenesis

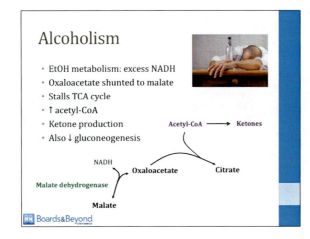

Urinary Ketones

- Normally no ketones in urine
  - Any produced → utilized
- Elevated urine ketones:
  - Poorly controlled diabetes (insufficient insulin)
  - DKA
  - Prolonged starvation
  - Alcoholism

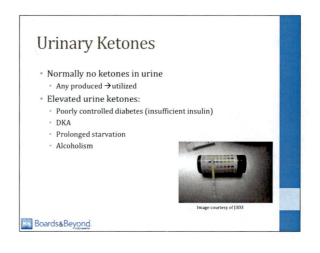

Ethanol Metabolism

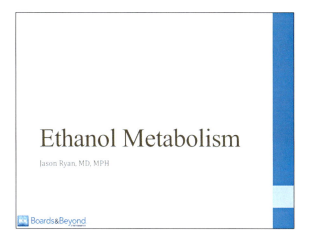

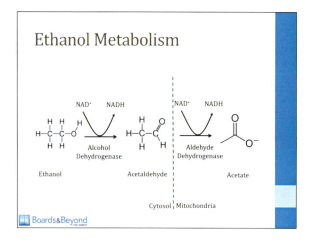

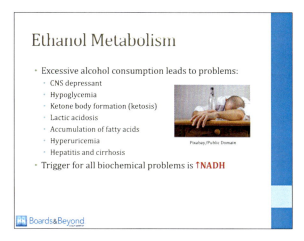

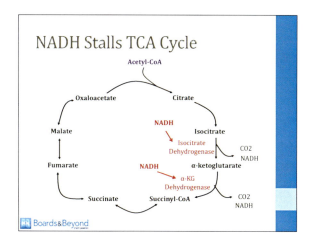

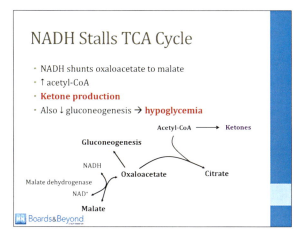

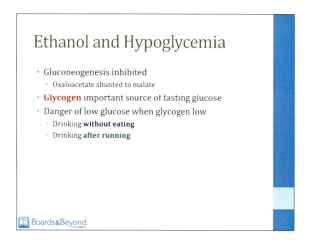

Ketones from Acetate

- Liver: Acetate → acetyl-CoA
- TCA cycle stalled due to high NADH
- Acetyl-CoA → ketones

Ketosis from Ethanol

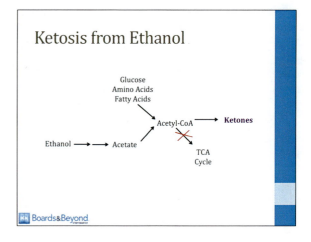

Lactic Acidosis

- Limited supply NAD⁺
- Depleted by EtOH metabolism
- Overwhelms electron transport
- Pyruvate shunted to lactate
- Regenerates NAD⁺

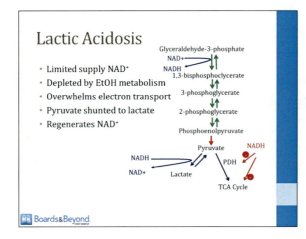

Accumulation of Fatty Acids

- High levels NADH stalls beta oxidation
  - Beta oxidation generates NADH (like TCA cycle)
  - Requires NAD+
  - Inhibited when NADH is high
- Result: ↓ FA breakdown

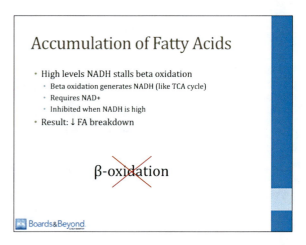

Accumulation of Fatty Acids

- Stalled TCA cycle → ↑ fatty acid synthesis

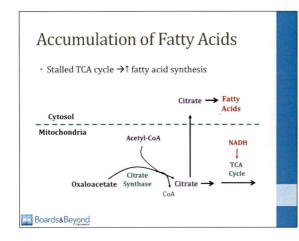

Accumulation of Fatty Acids

- Rate limiting step of fatty acid synthesis
- Favored when citrate high from slow TCA cycle

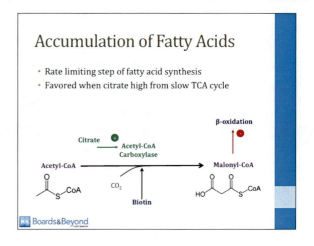

Accumulation of Fatty Acids

- **Malate** accumulation also contributes to FA levels
- Used to generate **NADPH**
- NADPH favors fatty acid synthesis

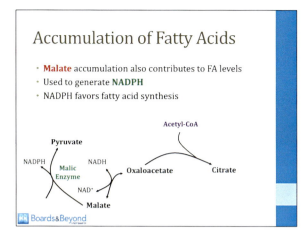

Accumulation of Fatty Acids

- **Fatty acid synthase**
- Uses carbons from acetyl CoA and malonyl CoA
- Creates 16 carbon fatty acid palmitate
- Requires **NADPH**

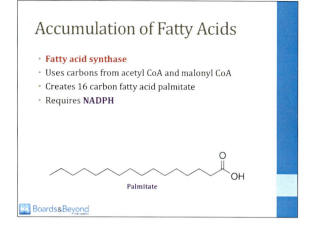

Fatty Acids and Ethanol

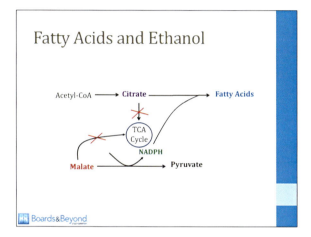

Glycerol

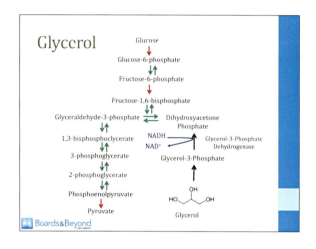

Fatty Liver

- Seen in alcoholism due to buildup of **triglycerides**

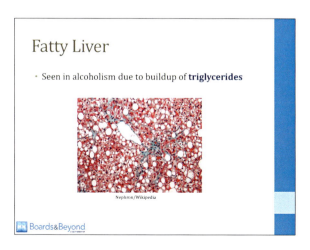

Uric Acid

- Urate and lactate excreted by proximal tubule
- ↑ lactate in plasma = ↓ excretion uric acid
- ↑ uric acid → gout attack
- Alcohol a well-described trigger for **gout**

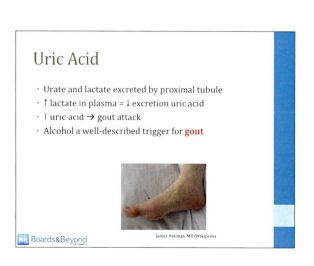

Hepatitis and Cirrhosis

- High NADH slows ethanol metabolism
- Result: **buildup of acetaldehyde**
- Toxic to liver cells
- Acute: Inflammation → Alcoholic hepatitis
- Chronic: Scar tissue → Cirrhosis

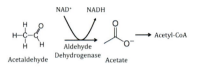 → Acetyl-CoA

Hepatitis and Cirrhosis

- **Microsomal ethanol-oxidizing system** (MEOS)
- Alternative pathway for ethanol
  - Normally metabolizes small amount of ethanol
  - Becomes important with excessive consumption
- Cytochrome P450-dependent pathway in **liver**
- Generates acetaldehyde and acetate
- Consumes NADPH and Oxygen
- Oxygen: generates free radicals
- NADPH: glutathione cannot be regenerated
  - Loss of protection from oxidative stress

Alcohol Dehydrogenase

- Zero order kinetics (constant rate)
- Also metabolizes methanol and ethylene glycol
- Inhibited by fomepizole (antizol)
  - Treatment for **methanol/ethylene glycol** intoxication

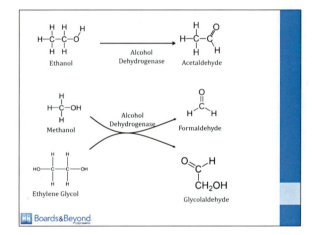

Aldehyde Dehydrogenase

- Inhibited by disulfiram (antabuse)
- Acetaldehyde accumulates
- Triggers catecholamine release
- **Sweating, flushing**, palpitations, nausea, vomiting

Alcohol Flushing

- Skin flushing when consuming alcohol
- Due to slow metabolism of acetaldehyde
- Common among Asian populations
  - Japan, China, Korea
  - Inherited deficiency aldehyde dehydrogenase 2 (ALDH2)
- Possible ↑risk esophageal and oropharyngeal cancer

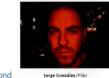

Jorge González/Flikr

Exercise and Starvation

Exercise and Starvation

Jason Ryan, MD, MPH

Exercise

- Rapidly depletes ATP in muscles
- Duration, intensity depends on other fuels
- Glycogen → Glucose → TCA cycle available **but slow**
- Short term needs met by creatine

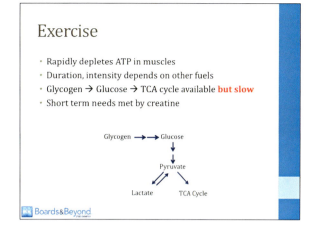

Creatine

- Present in muscles as **phosphocreatine**
- Source of phosphate groups
- Important for heart and muscles
- Can donate to ADP → ATP
- Reserve when ATP falls rapidly in early exercise

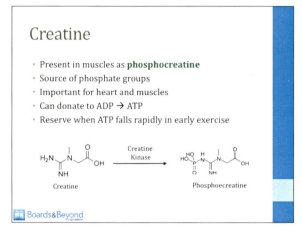

Creatinine

- Spontaneous conversion creatinine
- Amount of creatinine proportional to muscle mass
- Excreted by kidneys

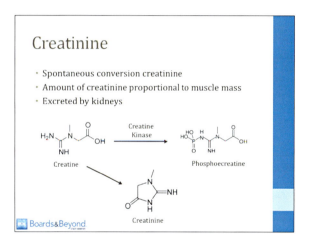

ATP and Creatine

- Consumed within seconds of exercise
- Used for short, intense exertion
  - Heavy lifting
  - Sprinting
- Exercise for longer time requires other pathways
- Slower metabolism
- Result: Exercise intensity diminishes with time

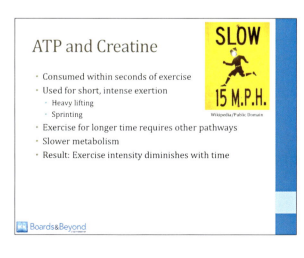

Calcium and Exercise

- Calcium release from muscles stimulates metabolism
- Activates glycogenolysis
- Activates TCA cycle

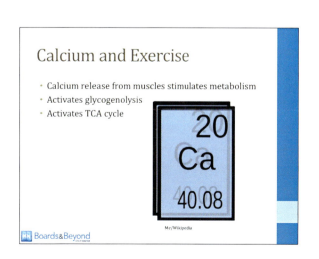

Calcium Activation
Glycogen Breakdown

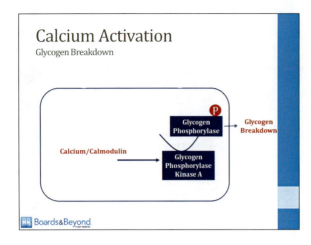

Calcium Activation
TCA Cycle

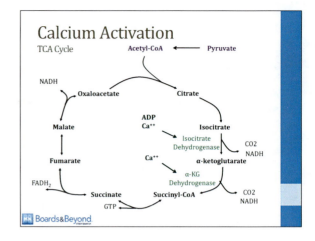

Types of Exercise

- Aerobic exercise
  - Long distance running
  - Co-ordinated effort by organ systems
  - Multiple potential sources of energy
- Anaerobic exercise
  - Sprinting, weight lifting
  - Purely a muscular effort
  - Blood vessels in muscles compressed during peak contraction
  - Muscle cells isolated from body
  - Muscle relies on it's own fuel stores

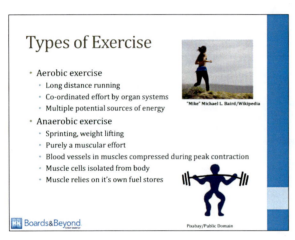

Anaerobic Exercise
40-yard sprint

- ATP and creatine phosphate (consumed in seconds)
- Glycogen
  - Metabolized to lactate (anaerobic metabolism)
  - TCA cycle too slow
- Fast pace cannot be maintained
  - Creatinine phosphate consumed
  - Lactate accumulates

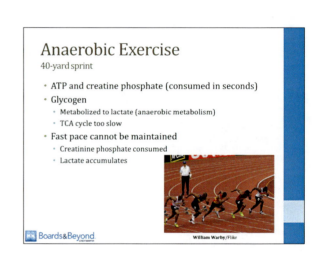

Moderate Aerobic Exercise
1-mile run

- ATP and creatine phosphate (consumed in seconds)
- Glycogen: metabolized to CO_2 (aerobic metabolism)
- Slower pace than sprint
  - Decrease lactate production
  - Allow time for TCA cycle and oxidative phosphorylation
- "Carbohydrate loading" by runners
  - Increases muscle glycogen content

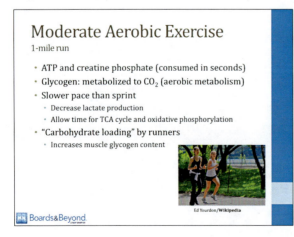

Intense Aerobic Exercise
Marathon

- Co-operation between muscle, liver, adipose tissue
- ATP and creatine phosphate (consumed in seconds)
- Muscle glycogen: metabolized to CO_2
- Liver glycogen: Assists muscles → produces glucose
- Often all glycogen consumed during race
- Conversion to metabolism of fatty acids
  - Slower process
  - Maximum speed of running reduced
- Elite runners condition to use glycogen/fatty acids

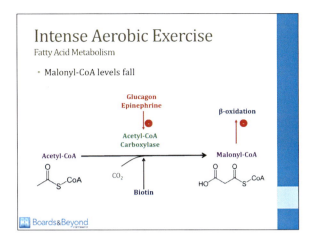
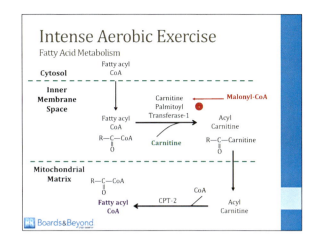
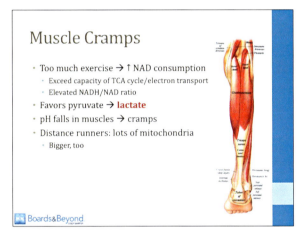
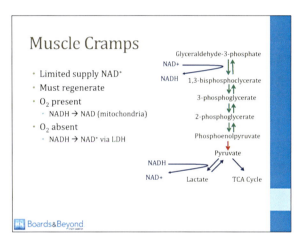
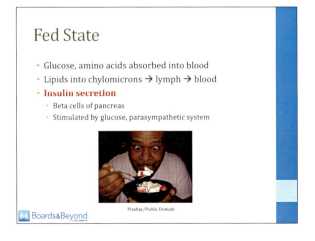
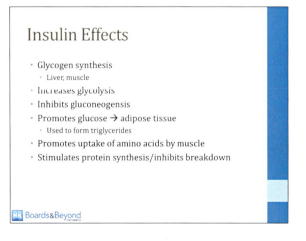

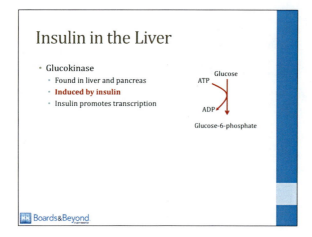
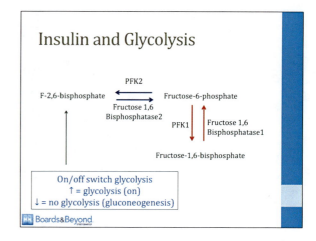
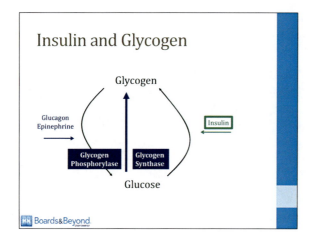
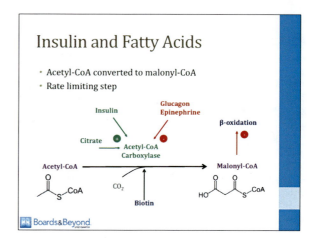
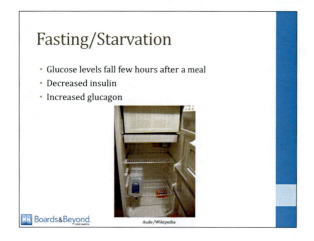
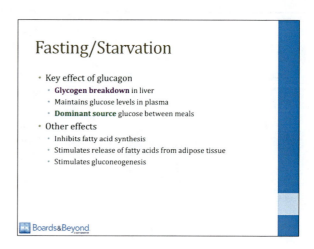

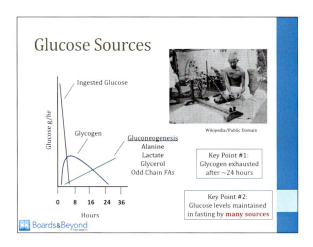
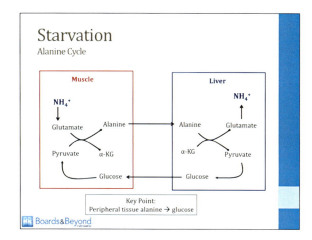
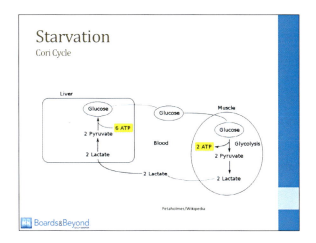
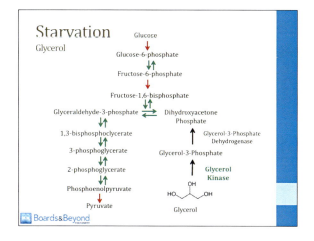

Starvation
Odd Chain Fatty Acids

- β-oxidation proceeds until 3 carbons remain
- Propionyl-CoA → Succinyl-CoA → TCA cycle
- Key point: Only odd chain FA → **glucose**

Starvation
Fuel Sources of Tissues

- Glycolysis slows (low insulin levels)
- Less glucose utilized by muscle/liver
- Shift to fatty acid beta oxidation for fuel
- Spares glucose and **maintains glucose levels**

Malnutrition

- Kwashiorkor
  - Inadequate protein intake
  - Hypoalbuminemia → **edema**
  - Swollen legs, abdomen

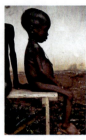

Malnutrition

- Marasmus
  - Inadequate energy intake
  - Insufficient **total calories**
  - Kwashiorkor without edema
  - Muscle, fat wasting

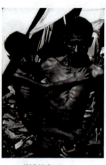

Hypoglycemia in Children

- Occurs with metabolic disorders
- **Glycogen storage diseases**
  - Hypoglycemia
  - Ketosis
  - Usually after overnight fast
- **Hereditary fructose intolerance**
  - Deficiency of aldolase B
  - Build-up of fructose 1-phosphate
  - Depletion of ATP
  - Usually a baby just weaned from breast milk

Hypoketotic Hypoglycemia

- Lack of ketones in setting of ↓ glucose during fasting
- Occurs in **beta oxidation disorders**
  - FFA → beta oxidation → ketones (beta oxidation)
  - Tissues overuse glucose → hypoglycemia

Hypoketotic Hypoglycemia

- **Carnitine deficiency**
  - Low serum **carnitine** and **acylcarnitine** levels
- **MCAD deficiency**
  - Medium chain acyl-CoA dehydrogenase
  - Dicarboxylic acids 6-10 carbons in urine
  - **High acylcarnitine levels**

Inborn Errors of Metabolism

Inborn Errors of Metabolism

Jason Ryan, MD, MPH

Inborn Errors in Metabolism

- Defects in metabolic pathways
- Often present in newborn period
- Often non-specific features:
  - Failure to thrive, hypotonia
- Lab findings suggest diagnosis:
  - Hypoglycemia
  - Ketosis
  - Hyperammonemia
  - Lactic acidosis

Newborn Hypoglycemia

- Glycogen storage diseases
- Galactosemia
- Hereditary fructose intolerance
- Organic acidemias
- Disorders of fatty acid metabolism

Glucose

Glycogen Storage Diseases

- Some have **no hypoglycemia**
  - Only affect muscles
  - McArdle's Disease (type V)
  - Pompe's Disease (type II)
- Hypoglycemia seen in others
  - Von Gierke's Disease (Type I)
  - Cori's Disease (Type III)

Glycogen Storage Diseases

- Fasting hypoglycemia
  - Hours after eating
  - Not in post-prandial period
- **Ketosis**
  - Absence of glucose during fasting
  - Fatty acid breakdown (NOT a fatty acid disorder)
  - Ketone synthesis
- Hepatomegaly
  - Glycogen buildup in liver

Glycogen Storage Diseases

- Von Gierke's Disease (Type I)
  - Severe hypoglycemia
  - Lactic acidosis
- Cori's Disease (Type III)
  - Gluconeogenesis intact
  - Mild hypoglycemia
  - No lactic acidosis

Cori Cycle

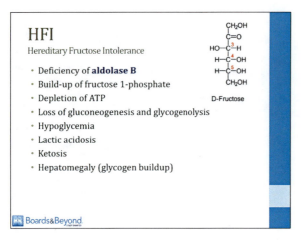
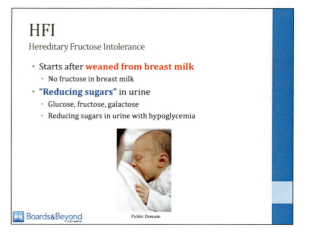
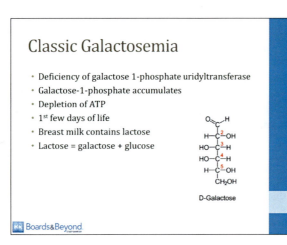
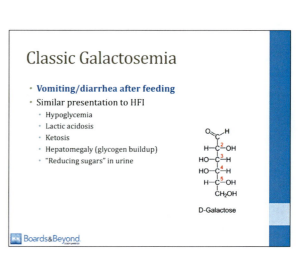
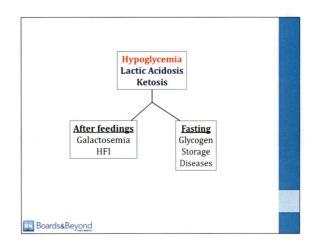
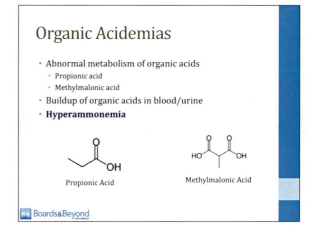

Succinyl-CoA

- Common pathway to TCA cycle
- Many substances metabolized to propionyl-CoA
- Propionyl-CoA → Methylmalonyl-CoA

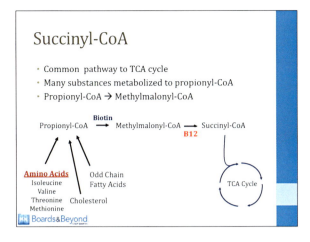

Organic Acidemias

- Onset in newborn period (weeks-months)
- Poor feeding, vomiting, hypotonia, lethargy
- Hypoglycemia → ketosis
  - Complex mechanism
  - Liver damage → ↓ gluconeogenesis
- Anion gap metabolic acidosis
- **Hyperammonemia**
- **Elevated urine/plasma organic acids**

Propionic Acidemia

- Deficiency of **propionyl-CoA carboxylase**

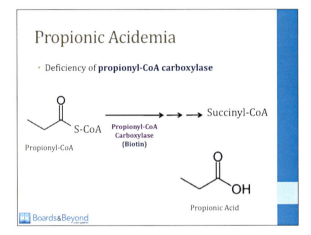

Methylmalonic Acidemia

- Deficiency of **methylmalonyl-CoA mutase**

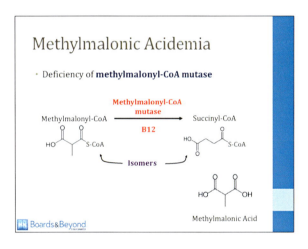

Maple Syrup Urine Disease

- Branched chain amino acid disorder
- Deficiency of **α-ketoacid dehydrogenase**
  - Multi-subunit complex
  - Cofactors: Thiamine, lipoic acid
- Amino acids and α-ketoacids in plasma/urine
- α-ketoacid of isoleucine gives urine sweet smell

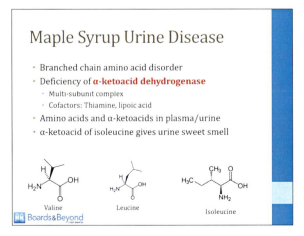

Fatty Acid Disorders

- Carnitine deficiency
- MCAD deficiency
  - Medium-chain-acyl-CoA dehydrogenase
  - Beta oxidation enzyme
- Both cause **hypoketotic hypoglycemia** when fasting
  - Lack of fatty acid breakdown → low ketone bodies
  - Overutilization of glucose → hypoglycemia
  - Lack of acetyl-CoA for gluconeogenesis

Fatty Acid Disorders

- Symptoms with fasting or illness
- Usually 3 months to 2 years
  - Frequent feedings < 3months prevent fasting
- Failure to thrive, altered consciousness, hypotonia
- Hepatomegaly
- Cardiomegaly
- **Hypoketotic hypoglycemia**

Primary Carnitine Deficiency

- Carnitine necessary for carnitine shuttle
  - Links with fatty acids forming acylcarnitine
  - Moves fatty acids into mitochondria for metabolism
- Muscle weakness, cardiomyopathy
- **Low carnitine and acylcarnitine levels**

Acyl-CoA + Carnitine → Acylcarnitine

MCAD Deficiency
Medium Chain Acyl-CoA Dehydrogenase

- Poor oxidation 6-10 carbon fatty acids
- **Dicarboxylic acids** 6-10 carbons in urine
  - Seen when beta oxidation impaired
- **High acylcarnitine levels**

Dicarboxylic Acid

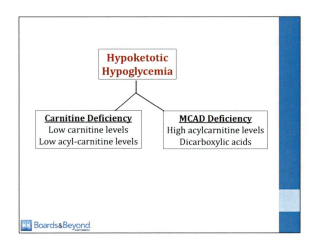

Hypoketotic Hypoglycemia

Carnitine Deficiency
Low carnitine levels
Low acyl-carnitine levels

MCAD Deficiency
High acylcarnitine levels
Dicarboxylic acids

Urea Cycle Disorders

- Onset in newborn period (first 24 to 48 hours)
- Feeding → protein load → symptoms
- Poor feeding, vomiting, lethargy
- May lead to seizures
- Lab tests: **Isolated severe hyperammonemia**
  - Normal < 50 mcg/dl
  - Urea disorder may be > 1000
- No other major metabolic derangements

OTC Deficiency
Ornithine transcarbamylase deficiency

- Most common urea cycle disorder
- ↑ carbamoyl phosphate
- ↑ orotic acid (derived from carbamoyl phosphate)

NH_4^+ → Carbamoyl Phosphate —Ornithine Transcarbamylase→ Urea Cycle

Glutamine → Carbamoyl Phosphate → Orotic Acid → Pyrimidines (U, C, T)

Pyrimidine Synthesis

Orotic Aciduria

- Disorder of pyrimidine synthesis
- Also has orotic aciduria
- **Normal ammonia levels**
- No somnolence, seizures
- Major features: Megaloblastic anemia, poor growth

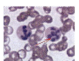
Megaloblastic Anemia

Mitochondrial Disorders

- Inborn errors of metabolism
- Loss of ability to metabolize pyruvate → acetyl CoA
- All cause **severe lactic acidosis**
- All cause **elevated alanine** (amino acid)
  - Pyruvate shunted to alanine and lactate
- Pyruvate dehydrogenase complex deficiency

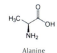
Alanine

Pyruvate

- End product of glycolysis

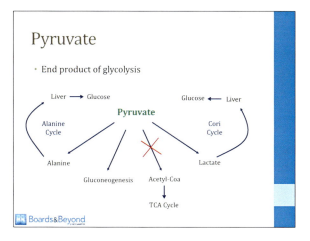

PDH Complex Deficiency
Pyruvate Dehydrogenase

- Pyruvate shunted to alanine, lactate
- Key findings (infancy):
  - Poor feeding
  - Growth failure
  - Developmental delays
- Labs:
  - Elevated alanine
  - Lactic acidosis
  - No hypoglycemia

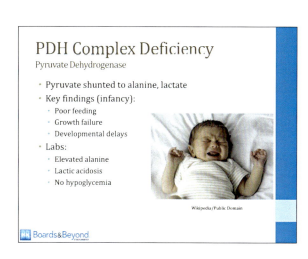

Wikipedia/Public Domain

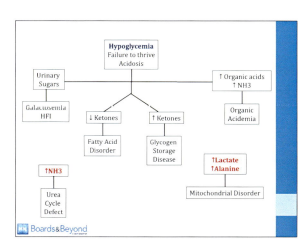

Amino Acids

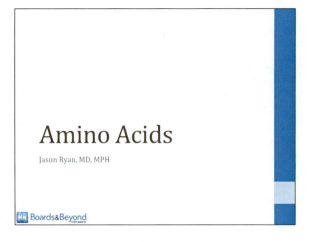

Amino Acids
Jason Ryan, MD, MPH

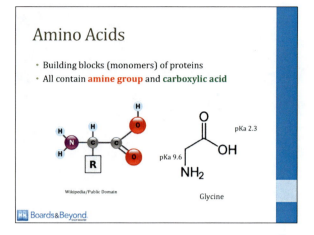

Amino Acids
- Building blocks (monomers) of proteins
- All contain **amine group** and **carboxylic acid**

Glycine — pKa 2.3, pKa 9.6

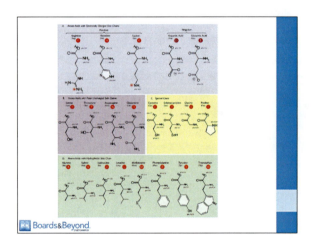

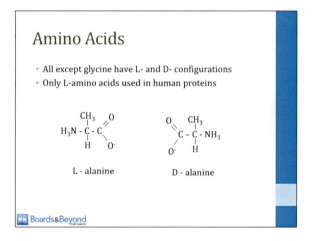

Amino Acids
- All except glycine have L- and D- configurations
- Only L-amino acids used in human proteins

L - alanine   D - alanine

pKa
log acid dissociation constant

$$HA \leftrightarrow A^- + H^+$$

$$pH = pKa + \log \frac{[A^-]}{[HA]}$$

$$pKa = pH - \log \frac{[A^-]}{[HA]}$$

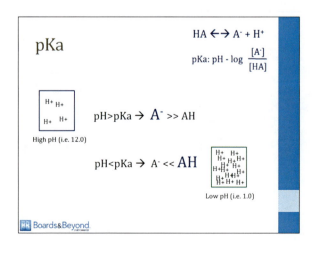

pKa

$$HA \leftrightarrow A^- + H^+$$

$$pKa: pH - \log \frac{[A^-]}{[HA]}$$

High pH (i.e. 12.0)   pH > pKa → $A^- \gg AH$

pH < pKa → $A^- \ll AH$ Low pH (i.e. 1.0)

pKa

- Acetic acid (C_2O_2H) pKa = 4.75

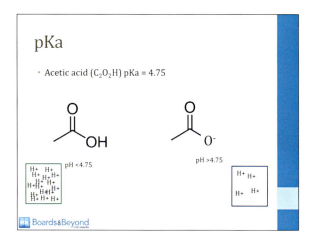

pKa

- Ammonia (NH_3) pKa = 9.4

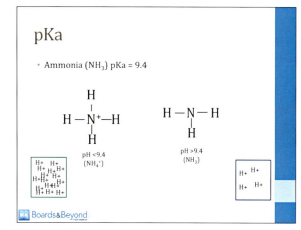

pKa

- Amino acids: multiple acid-base regions
- Each has different pKa

R–COOH → R–COO⁻ + H⁺ Usually low pKa < 4.0
At normal pH (7.4): COO-

R–NH_3^+ → R–NH_2 + H⁺ Usually high pKa > 9.0
At normal pH (7.4): NH_3

pKa

- Some side chains have pKa (3 pKa values!)

Lysine
- NH_3^+ pKa=10.53
- H_3N^+ pKa=8.95
- COO⁻ pKa=2.18

Titration Curves

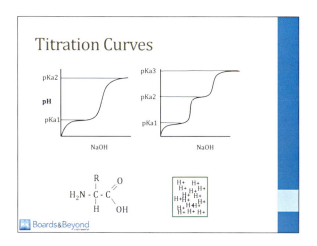

Charge at Normal pH

- Normal plasma pH=7.4
- AA charge (+/-) depends on pKa values

Glycine
- COO⁻ pKa=2.2
- NH_3^+ pKa=9.6

Charge at Normal pH

Arginine

Basic Amino Acids

Arginine
*most basic AA

Lysine

Both +1 charge at normal pH
Remove 1H⁺ from solution
Raise pH (basic)

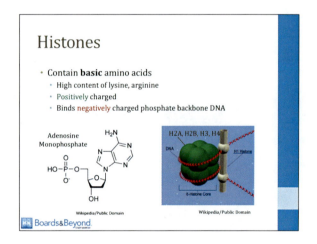
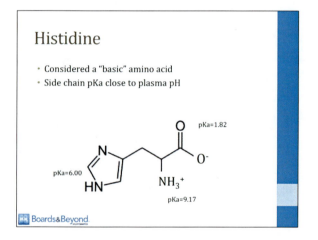

Histones

- Contain **basic** amino acids
  - High content of lysine, arginine
  - Positively charged
  - Binds negatively charged phosphate backbone DNA

Histidine

- Considered a "basic" amino acid
- Side chain pKa close to plasma pH

Acidic Amino Acids

Aspartate

Glutamate

Hydrophobic Amino Acids

Proline, Methionine, Alanine, Glycine
Tryptophan, Leucine, Phenylalanine
Valine, Isoleucine

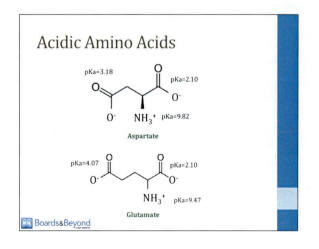
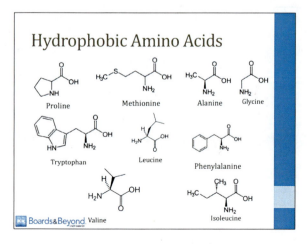

Sickle Cell Anemia

- Exchange of polar **glutamate** for nonpolar **valine** in hemoglobin protein

Proline

- Rigid structure (ring) formed from amino group and side chain
- Used in collagen

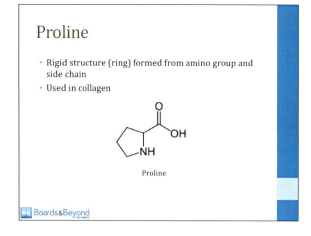

Essential Amino Acids

- **Nine** amino acids must be supplied by diet
- Cannot be synthesized de novo by cells

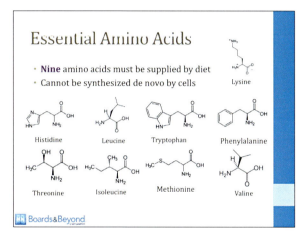

Glucogenic vs. Ketogenic

- Glucogenic amino acids:
  - Can be converted to pyruvate or TCA cycle intermediates
  - Can become glucose via gluconeogenesis
- Ketogenic amino acids
  - Convert to ketone bodies and acetyl CoA
  - Cannot become glucose
- Most amino acids are either:
  - Glucogenic
  - Glucogenic and ketogenic

Glucogenic vs. Ketogenic

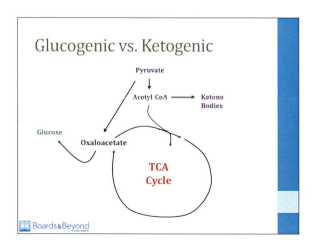

Ketogenic Amino Acids

*both essential

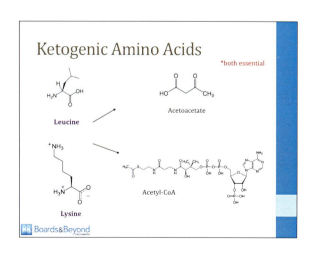

Phenylalanine and Tyrosine

Phenylalanine and Tyrosine

- Key amino acids for synthesis of:
  - Dopamine, Norepinephrine, Epinephrine
  - Thyroid hormone, Melanin
- Metabolism: several important vitamins/cofactors
- Three metabolic disorders:
  - Phenylketonuria (PKU)
  - Albinism
  - Alkaptonuria

Phenylalanine

- Alanine with a phenyl group added

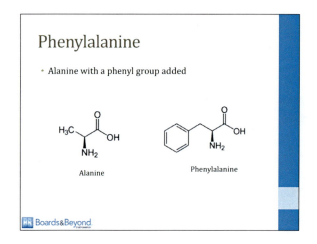

Phenylalanine

- Converted to tyrosine (non-essential amino acid)

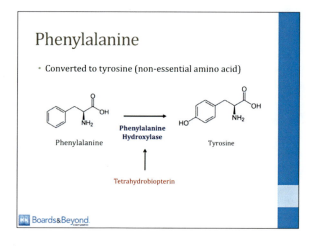

Tetrahydrobiopterin
BH4

- Cofactor for phenylalanine metabolism

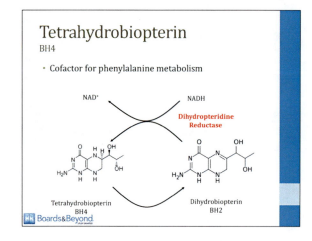

Phenylalanine

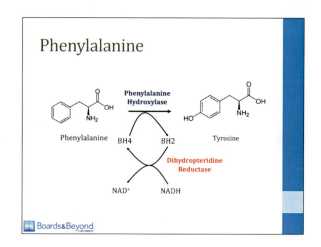

Phenylketonuria
PKU

- Deficiency of phenylalanine hydroxylase activity
  - Defective enzyme (classic PKU)
  - Defective/deficient BH4 cofactor
- Most common inborn error of metabolism
- Accumulation of phenylalanine
- Deficiency of tyrosine (sometimes low normal)

Phenylketonuria
PKU

- Metabolites of phenylalanine → toxicity

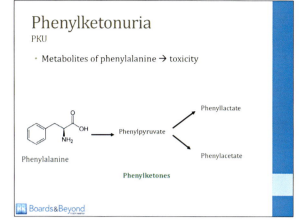

Phenylketones

Phenylketonuria
Signs and Symptoms

- Musty smell in urine from phenylalanine metabolites
- CNS Symptoms
  - Intellectual disability
  - Seizures
  - Tremor
- Pale skin, fair hair, blue eyes
  - Lack of tyrosine conversion to melanin

Phenylketonuria
Treatment

- Dietary modification
  - **Restriction of phenylalanine**
  - Found in most proteins (essential amino acid)
  - Synthetic amino acids mixtures use for food
  - Phenylalanine level monitored
  - **No aspartame** (Equal/NutraSweet)
  - **Tyrosine becomes essential**

Aspartame (aspartate + phenylalanine)

Phenylketonuria

- Maternal PKU
  - Occurs in **women with PKU** who consume phenylalanine
  - High levels of phenylalanine acts as a **teratogen**
  - Baby born with microcephaly, congenital heart defects

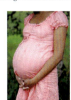

Øyvind Holmstad/Wikipedia

Phenylketonuria
Screening

- Newborn measurement of phenylalanine level
- Done 2-3 days after birth
  - Maternal enzymes may normalize levels at birth

Achoubey/Wikipedia

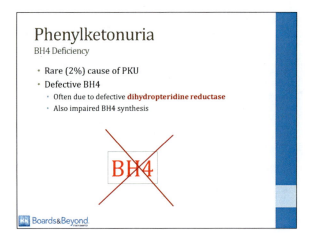
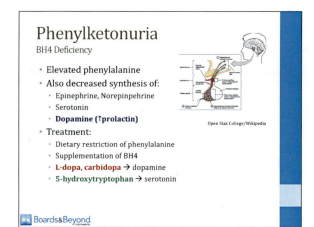
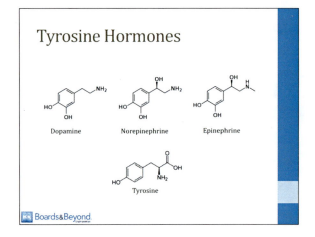
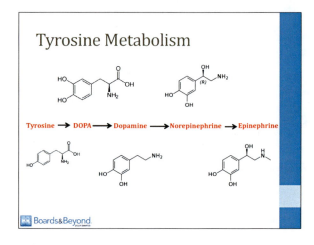
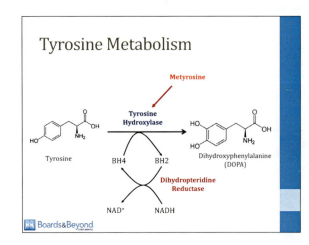
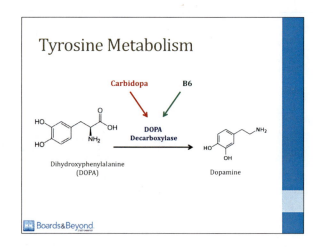

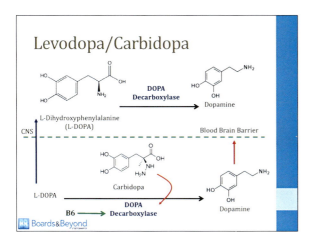
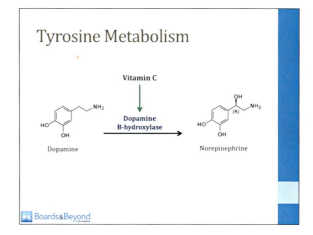
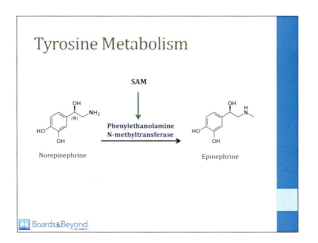
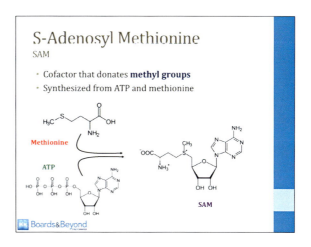
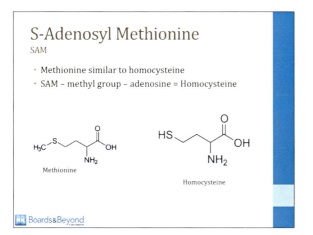
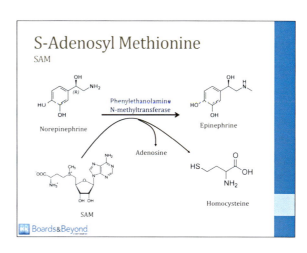

S-Adenosyl Methionine
SAM

- Need to regenerate methionine to maintain SAM
- Requires folate and vitamin B12

S-Adenosyl Methionine
SAM

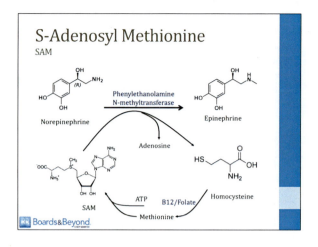

Tyrosine Metabolism

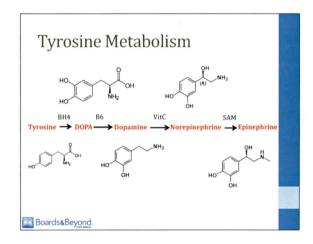

Tyrosine → DOPA → Dopamine → Norepinephrine → Epinephrine
(BH4, B6, VitC, SAM)

Thyroxine (T4)

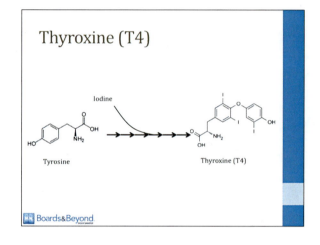

Melanin

- Pigment in skin, hair, eyes
- Synthesized by melanocytes
- Polymer of repeating units made from tyrosine

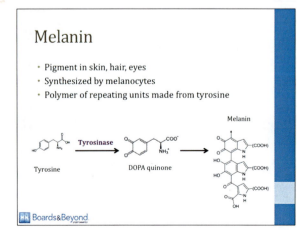

Oculocutaneous albinism
(OCA)

- Most commonly from deficiency of:
  - Tyrosinase (OCA Type I)
  - Tyrosine transporters (OCA Type II)
- Decreased/absent melanin
- Pale skin, blond hair, blue eyes
- ↑ risk of **sunburns**
- ↑ risk of **skin cancer**

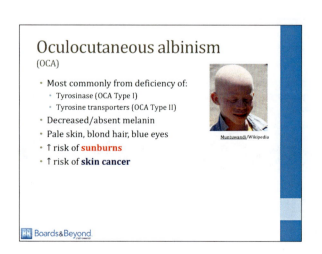

Oculocutaneous albinism
(OCA)

- Seen in **Chediak-Higashi Syndrome**
  - Immunodeficiency
  - OCA Type II: Transporter defect
- Ocular albinism:
  - Rare variant, blue eyes only

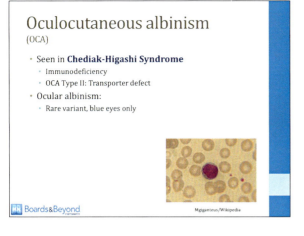

Tyrosine Breakdown

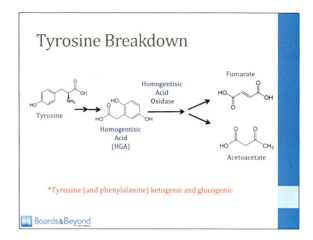

*Tyrosine (and phenylalanine) ketogenic and glucogenic

Alkaptonuria
Ochronosis

- Deficiency of **homogentisic acid oxidase**
- Autosomal recessive
- ↑ homogentisic acid
- Polymerization → dark pigment
- Pigment deposited in connective tissue (ochronosis)

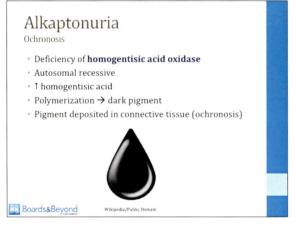

Alkaptonuria
Ochronosis

- Classic finding: dark urine **when left standing**
  - Fresh urine normal → polymerization
- **Arthritis** (large joints: knees, hips)
  - Severe arthritis may be crippling
- **Black pigment** in cartilage, joints
- Classic X-ray finding: calcification intervertebral discs
- Urine discoloration in infancy
- Other symptoms later in life (20-30 years)

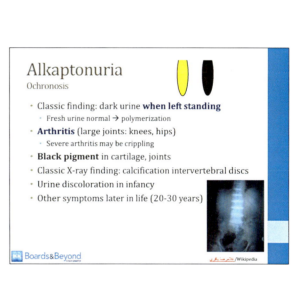

Alkaptonuria
Ochronosis

- Diagnosis
  - **Elevated HGA** in urine/plasma
- Treatment:
  - Dietary restriction (tyrosine and phenylalanine)

Catecholamine Breakdown

- Monoamines: Dopamine, norepinephrine, epinephrine
- Degradation via two enzymes:
  - **Monamine oxidase (MAO):** Amine → COOH
  - **Catechol-O-methyltransferase (COMT):** Methyl to oxygen
- Epi, Norepi → Vanillymandelic acid (VMA)
- Dopamine → Homovanillic acid (HVA)
- HVA and VMA excreted in urine

Tyrosine Hormones

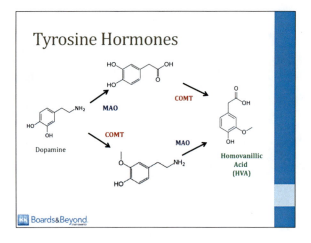

Tyrosine Hormones

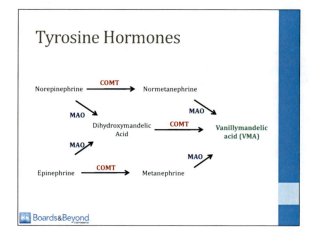

Pheochromocytoma

- Tumor generating catecholamines
- Majority of metabolism is intratumoral
- **Metanephrines** often measured for diagnosis
    - Metanephrine and normetanephrine
    - 24hour urine collection
- Older test: 24 hour collection of VMA

Pharmacology

- **Parkinson's**
    - Selegiline: MAO-b inhibitor
    - Entacapone, tolacpone: COMT inhibitors
    - ↑ dopamine levels
- **Depression**
    - MAO inhibitors (Tranylcypromine, Phenelzine)
    - ↑ dopamine, NE, serotonin levels

Tyramine

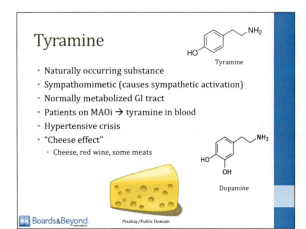

- Naturally occurring substance
- Sympathomimetic (causes sympathetic activation)
- Normally metabolized GI tract
- Patients on MAOi → tyramine in blood
- Hypertensive crisis
- "Cheese effect"
    - Cheese, red wine, some meats

Other Amino Acids

Jason Ryan, MD, MPH

Amino Acids

- Tryptophan → Niacin, serotonin, melatonin
- Histidine → Histamine
- Glycine → Heme
- Arginine → Creatine, urea, nitric oxide
- Glutamate → GABA
- Branched chain amino acids (Maple syrup urine)
- Homocysteine (homocystinuria)
- Cysteine (cystinuria)

Tryptophan

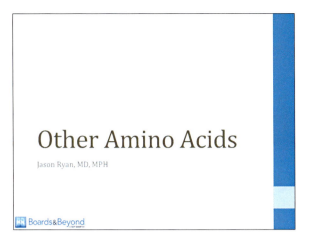

Tryptophan

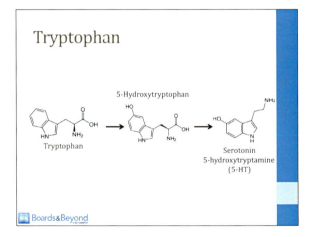

Carcinoid Syndrome

- Caused by **GI tumors** that secrete serotonin
- Altered **tryptophan metabolism**
  - Normally ~1% tryptophan → serotonin
  - Up to 70% in patients with carcinoid syndrome
  - **Tryptophan deficiency (pellagra)** reported
- Serotonin effects
  - Diarrhea (serotonin stimulates GI motility)
  - ↑ fibroblast growth and fibrogenesis → valvular lesions
  - Flushing (other mediators also)

Serotonin Breakdown

- Metabolism via **monoamine oxidase**
  - Same enzyme: dopamine/epinephrine/norepinephrine
- **MAO Inhibitors** used in depression (↑serotonin)
- **↑ Urinary 5-HIAA** in carcinoid syndrome

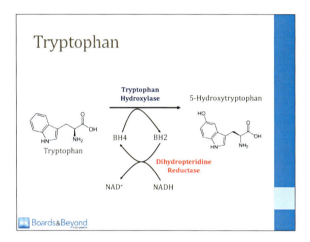

Tryptophan

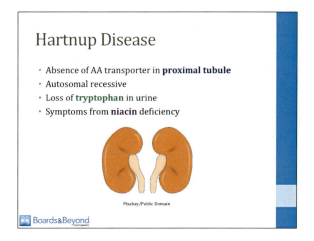

Tryptophan

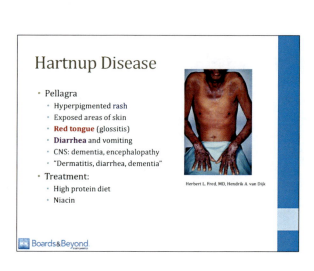

Hartnup Disease

- Absence of AA transporter in **proximal tubule**
- Autosomal recessive
- Loss of **tryptophan** in urine
- Symptoms from **niacin** deficiency

Hartnup Disease

- Pellagra
  - Hyperpigmented **rash**
  - Exposed areas of skin
  - **Red tongue** (glossitis)
  - **Diarrhea** and vomiting
  - CNS: dementia, encephalopathy
  - "Dermatitis, diarrhea, dementia"
- Treatment:
  - High protein diet
  - Niacin

Histidine

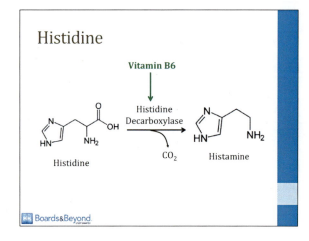

Glycine

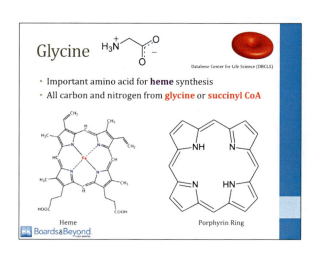

- Important amino acid for **heme** synthesis
- All carbon and nitrogen from **glycine** or **succinyl CoA**

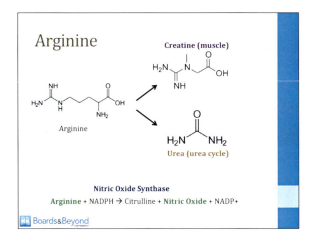

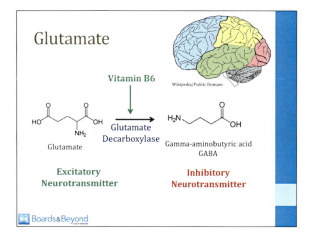

Branched Chain Amino Acids

- Essential amino acids
- Primarily metabolized by muscle cells
- Metabolism depends on **α-ketoacid dehydrogenase**
  - Branched-chain α-ketoacid dehydrogenase complex (BCKDC)
  - Similar to pyruvate dehydrogenase complex
  - E1, E2, E3 subunits
  - Cofactors: Thiamine, lipoic acid

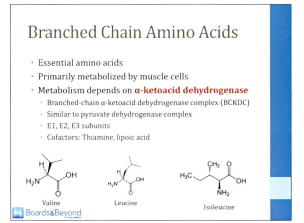

Branched Chain Amino Acids

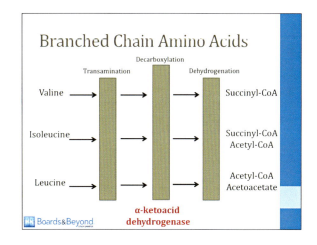

Maple Syrup Urine Disease

- Deficiency of **α-ketoacid dehydrogenase**
- Autosomal recessive
- Five phenotypes
- Classic MSUD most common (E1, E2, E3 deficiency)
- ↑ branched chain AA's and α-ketoacids in plasma
- α-ketoacid of isoleucine gives urine sweet smell

Maple Syrup Urine Disease

- **Neurotoxicity** is main problem MSUD
- Primarily due to accumulation of **leucine**: "leucinosis"
- Classic MSUD occurs in 1st few days of life
- Lethargy and irritability
- Apnea, seizures
- Signs of cerebral edema

Maple Syrup Urine Disease

- Diagnosis:
  - Elevated **branched chain amino acid** levels in plasma
    - Valine, leucine, isoleucine
- Treatment:
  - **Dietary restriction** of branched-chain amino acids
  - Monitoring plasma amino acid concentrations
  - Thiamine supplementation

Homocysteine

- **Homocysteine**, **cysteine**, and **methionine** related
- Methionine: essential
- Cysteine: non-essential
  - Synthesized from methionine
- Homocysteine: non-standard
- Transsulfuration pathway
  - Methionine → homocysteine → cysteine

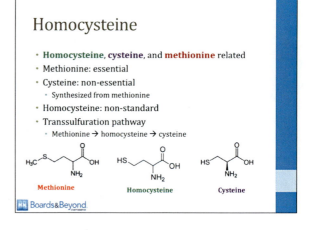

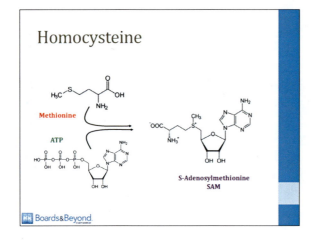

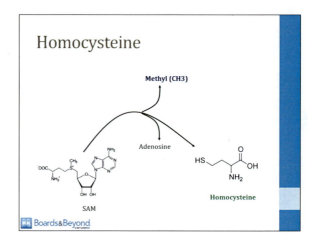

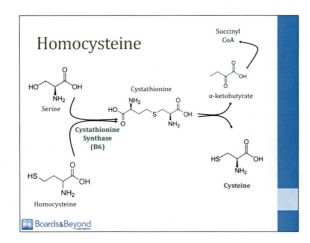

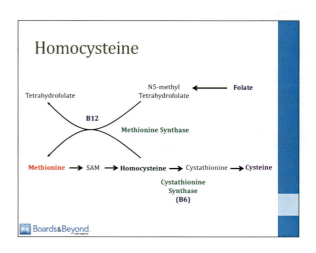

Homocysteine Levels

- Normal: 5-15 micromoles/liter
- Mild-moderate elevations:
  - Can be caused by vitamin deficiencies: B12/folate, B6
  - May be associated with ↑ risk CV disease
  - No data on lowering levels to lower risk

Homocystinuria

- Severe hyperhomocysteinemia: >100micromoles/liter
- Defects in homocysteine metabolism enzymes
- Autosomal recessive disorders

Homocystinuria

- Common symptoms (mechanisms unclear)
  - **Lens** dislocation
  - Long limbs, chest deformities
  - Osteoporosis in childhood
  - **Blood clots**
  - Early atherosclerosis (stroke, MI)

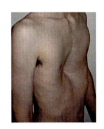

Ahellwig/Wikipedia

Homocystinuria

- Classic homocystinuria:
  - **Cystathionine β synthase (CBS)** deficiency
- Dietary treatment:
  - Avoid **methionine**
  - Increase cysteine (now essential)
  - Vitamin B6 supplementation (some patients "B6 responders")

Homocysteine Elevations
Less common causes

- Methionine synthase deficiency
- Defective metabolism folate/B12
  - MTHFR gene mutations

Homocysteine

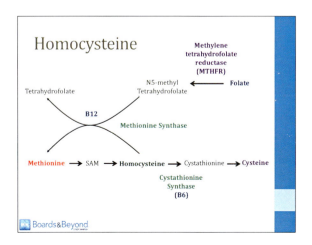

Cystinuria

- Cystine: Two cysteine molecules linked together
- Cystinuria: autosomal recessive disorder
- ↓ reabsorption cystine by proximal tubule of nephron
- Main problem: **kidney stones**
- Prevention: **methionine** free diet

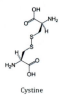

Cystine

Ammonia

Ammonia

Jason Ryan, MD, MPH

Amino Acid Breakdown

- No storage form of amino acids
- Unused amino acids broken down
- Amino group removed → NH_3 + α-keto acid

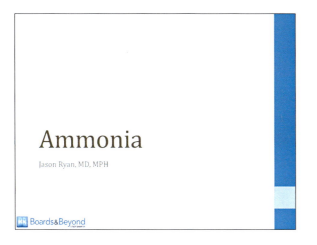

Ammonia

- Toxic to body
- Transferred to liver in a non-toxic structure
- Converted by liver to urea (non-toxic) for excretion

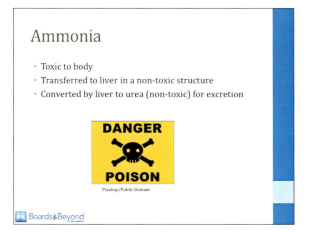

Amino Acid Breakdown

- Usual 1st step: removal of nitrogen by **transamination**
- Amino group passed to **glutamate**

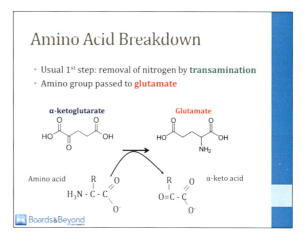

Aminotransferases

- Transfer nitrogen from amino acids to glutamate
- All require **vitamin B6** as cofactor
- Two used as liver function tests:
  - Alanine aminotransferase (ALT)
  - Aspartate aminotransferase (AST)

Aminotransferases

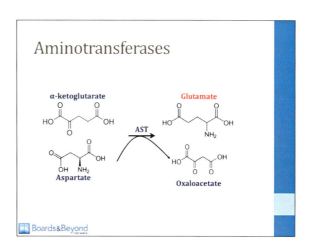

Glutamate

- Two methods for transfer of nitrogen from glutamate to liver for excretion in urea cycle
- #1: Glutamine synthesis
- #2: Alanine cycle

Glutamine

- Non-toxic
- Transfers nitrogen to liver for excretion
- Glutamine synthetase found in most tissues

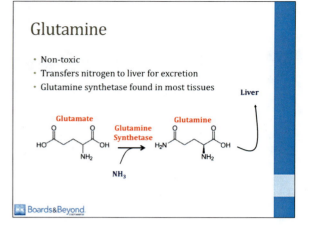

Glutamine

- In liver, glutamine converted back to glutamate

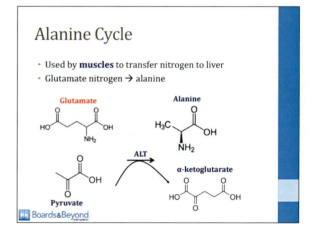

Alanine Cycle

- Used by **muscles** to transfer nitrogen to liver
- Glutamate nitrogen → alanine

Alanine Cycle

- Alanine to liver → pyruvate
- Nitrogen transferred back to glutamate

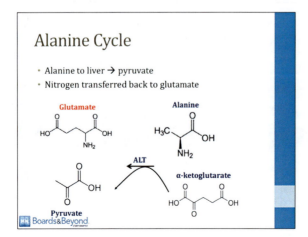

Alanine Cycle

- Nitrogen removed from glutamate

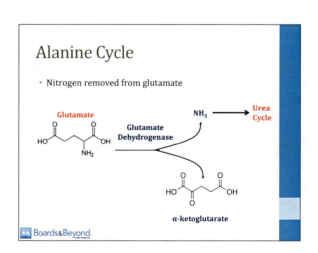

Alanine Cycle

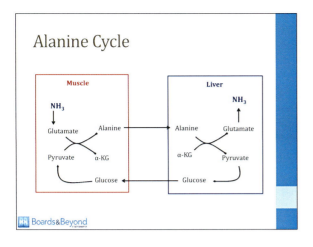

Mitochondrial Disorders

- Inborn errors of metabolism
- Often deficient metabolism of pyruvate
  - Pyruvate carboxylase deficiency
  - Pyruvate dehydrogenase deficiency
- Elevated **alanine** and lactate

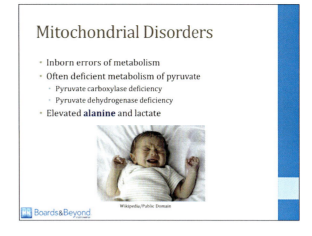

Urea Cycle

- Ammonia (NH_4^+) → Urea → Excretion in urine
- Urea synthesized from:
  - Ammonia
  - Carbon dioxide
  - Aspartate

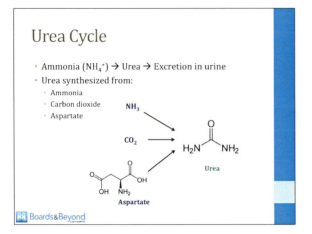

Urea Cycle

- First reaction (and 2nd) in mitochondria
- Rate limiting step

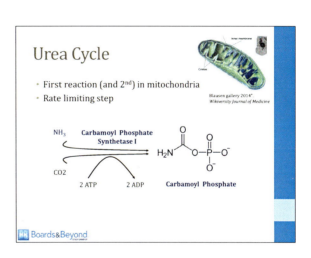

N-acetylglutamate

- Allosteric **activator**
- **Carbamoyl Phosphate Synthetase I**
- Enzyme will not function without this cofactor
- Synthesized from glutamate and acetyl CoA
- ↑ protein (fed state) → ↑ N-acetylglutamate
- Used to regulate urea cycle

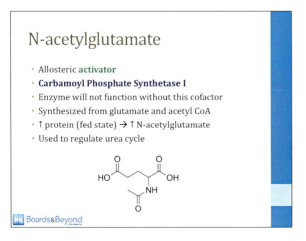

Pyrimidine Synthesis

- **Carbamoyl phosphate synthetase II**

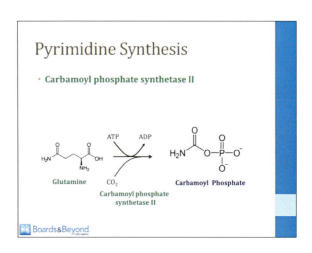

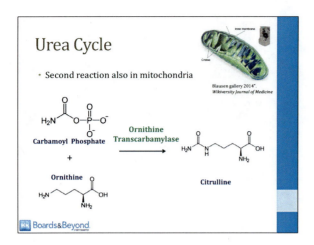
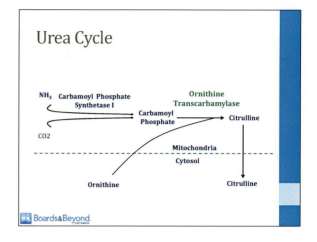
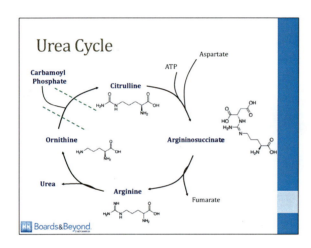
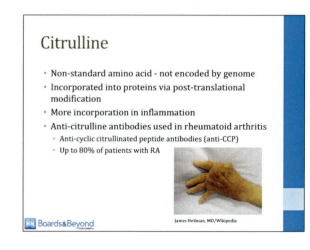
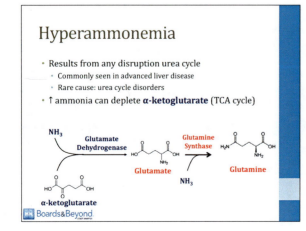
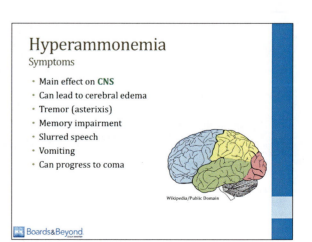

Hyperammonemia
Treatment

- Low protein diet ~~STEAK~~
- Lactulose
  - Synthetic disaccharide (laxative)
  - Colon breakdown by bacteria to fatty acids
  - Lowers colonic pH; favors formation of NH_4^+ over NH_3
  - NH_4^+ not absorbed → trapped in colon
  - Result: ↓plasma ammonia concentrations

Hyperammonemia
Treatment: Enzyme deficiencies only

- Ammonium Detoxicants
  - Sodium phenylbutyrate (oral)
  - Sodium phenylacetate-sodium benzoate (IV)
  - Conjugate with glutamine
  - Excreted in the urine → removal of nitrogen/ammonia
- Arginine supplementation
  - Urea cycle disorders make arginine essential

OTC Deficiency
Ornithine transcarbamylase deficiency

- Most common urea cycle disorder
- X linked recessive
- ↑ carbamoyl phosphate
- ↑ ammonia
- ↑ orotic acid (derived from carbamoyl phosphate)

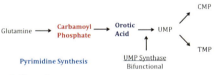

OTC Deficiency
Ornithine transcarbamylase deficiency

- Presents in infancy or childhood
  - Depends on severity of defect
  - If severe, occurs after first several feedings (protein)
- Symptoms from hyperammonemia
- Somnolence, poor feeding
- Seizures
- Vomiting, lethargy, coma

OTC Deficiency
Ornithine transcarbamylase deficiency

- Don't confuse with orotic aciduria
  - Disorder of pyrimidine synthesis
  - Also has orotic aciduria
  - OTC only: ↑ **ammonia levels** (urea cycle dysfunction)
  - Ammonia → encephalopathy (child with lethargy, coma)

Citrullinemia

- Deficiency of **argininosuccinate synthase**
- Elevated **citrulline**
- Low arginine
- Hyperammonemia

Other Urea Cycle Disorders

- Deficiencies of each enzyme described
- All autosomal recessive except OTC deficiency
- All cause **hyperammonemia**
- Build-up of urea cycle intermediates

B Vitamins

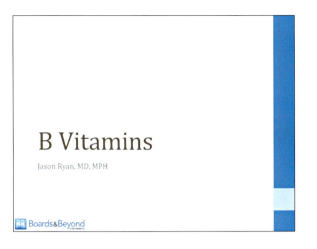

B Vitamins
Jason Ryan, MD, MPH

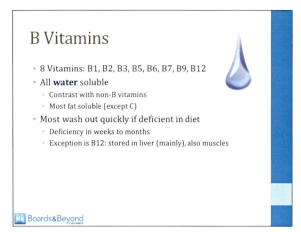

B Vitamins
- 8 Vitamins: B1, B2, B3, B5, B6, B7, B9, B12
- All **water** soluble
  - Contrast with non-B vitamins
  - Most fat soluble (except C)
- Most wash out quickly if deficient in diet
  - Deficiency in weeks to months
  - Exception is B12: stored in liver (mainly), also muscles

B Vitamins
- Used in many different metabolic pathways
- Deficiencies: greatest effect on rapidly growing tissues
- Common symptoms
  - Dermatitis (skin)
  - Glossitis (swelling/redness of tongue)
  - Diarrhea (GI tract)
  - Cheilitis (skin breakdown at corners of lips)

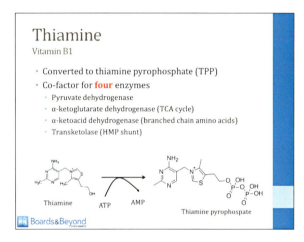

Thiamine
Vitamin B1
- Converted to thiamine pyrophosphate (TPP)
- Co-factor for **four** enzymes
  - Pyruvate dehydrogenase
  - α-ketoglutarate dehydrogenase (TCA cycle)
  - α-ketoacid dehydrogenase (branched chain amino acids)
  - Transketolase (HMP shunt)

Pyruvate

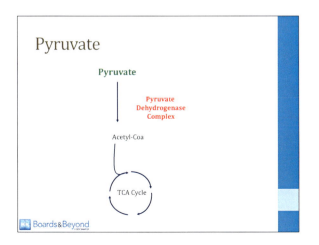

Pyruvate Dehydrogenase Complex
- Complex of 3 enzymes (E1, E2, E3)
  - Pyruvate dehydrogenase (E1)
- Requires 5 co-factors
  - Thiamine (B1)
  - FAD (B2)
  - NAD⁺ (B3)
  - Coenzyme A (B5)
  - Lipoic acid

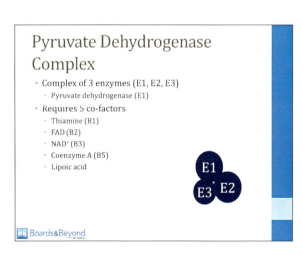

α-KG Dehydrogenase

- TCA cycle

α-ketoglutarate → Succinyl-CoA (via α-KG Dehydrogenase; CoA in, CO2 + NADH out)

Branched Chain Amino Acids

- Metabolism depends on **α-ketoacid dehydrogenase**
- Deficiency: **Maple Syrup Urine Disease**

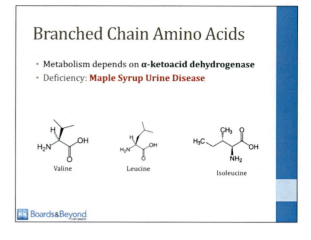

Valine, Leucine, Isoleucine

Transketolase
HMP Shunt

- Transfers a carbon unit to create F-6-phosphate
- **Wernicke-Korsakoff syndrome**
  - Abnormal transketolase may predispose
  - Affected individuals may have abnormal binding to thiamine

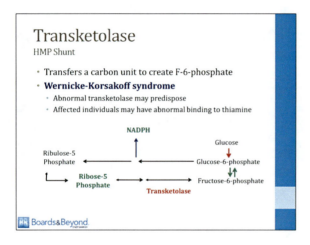

Thiamine Deficiency

- **Beriberi**
  - Underdeveloped areas
  - Dry type: polyneuritis, muscle weakness
  - Wet type: tachycardia, high-output heart failure, edema
- **Wernicke-Korsakoff syndrome**
  - Alcoholics (malnourished, poor absorption vitamins)
  - Confusion, confabulation
  - Ataxia
  - Ophthalmoplegia (blurry vision)

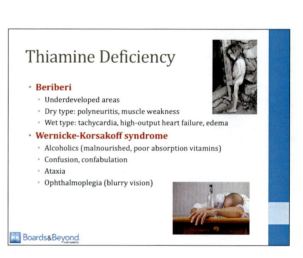

Thiamine and Glucose

- Malnourished patients: ↓glucose ↓thiamine
- If glucose given first → unable to metabolize
- Case reports of worsening Wernicke-Korsakoff

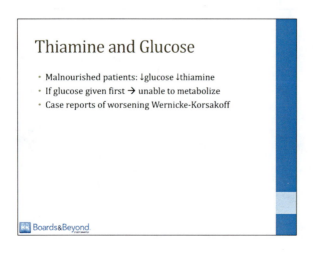

Riboflavin
Vitamin B2

- Added to adenosine → FAD
- Accepts 2 electrons → $FADH_2$
- FAD required by **dehydrogenases**
- **Electron transport chain**

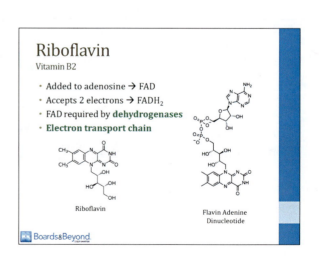

Riboflavin — Flavin Adenine Dinucleotide

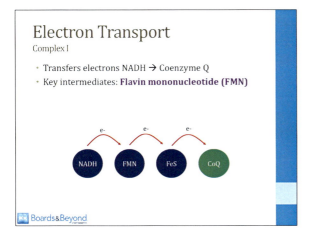
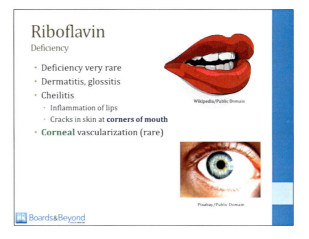
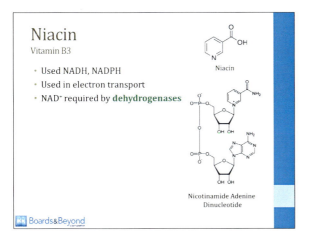
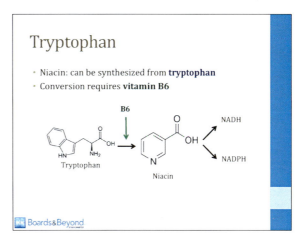
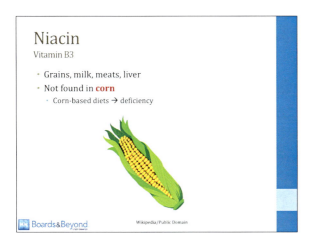
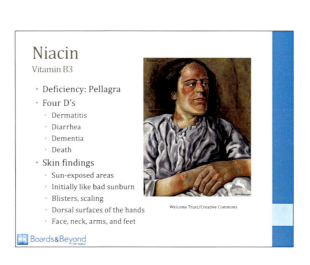

Niacin Deficiency

- **INH therapy** (tuberculosis)
  - INH → ↓B6 activity
  - ↓B6 activity → ↓Niacin (from tryptophan)
- Hartnup disease
- Carcinoid syndrome

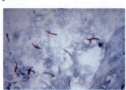

Hartnup Disease

- Absence of AA transporter in **proximal tubule**
- Autosomal recessive
- Loss of **tryptophan** in urine
- Symptoms from **niacin** deficiency

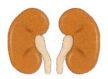

Carcinoid Syndrome

- Caused by **GI tumors** that secrete serotonin
  - Diarrhea, flushing, cardiac valve disease
- Altered **tryptophan metabolism**
  - Normally ~1% tryptophan → serotonin
  - Up to 70% in patients with carcinoid syndrome
  - **Tryptophan deficiency (pellagra)** reported

Niacin
Vitamin B3

- Also used to treat **hyperlipidemia**
- Direct effects on lipolysis (unrelated NAD/NADP)

Niacin Excess

- Facial **flushing**
  - Seen with niacin treatment for hyperlipidemia
  - Stimulates release of prostaglandins in skin
  - **Face** turns red, warm
  - Can blunt with **aspirin** (inhibits prostaglandin) prior to Niacin
  - Fades with time

Pantothenic Acid
Vitamin B5

- Used in **coenzyme A**
- CoA required by **dehydrogenases**/other enzymes

β-oxidation

- Step #1: Convert fatty acid to fatty acyl CoA

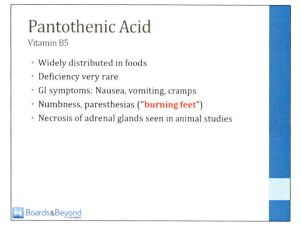

Pantothenic Acid
Vitamin B5

- Widely distributed in foods
- Deficiency very rare
- GI symptoms: Nausea, vomiting, cramps
- Numbness, paresthesias ("**burning feet**")
- Necrosis of adrenal glands seen in animal studies

Vitamin B6

- Three compounds
  - Pyridoxine (plants)
  - Pyridoxal, pyridoxamine (animals)
- All converted to **pyridoxal phosphate**

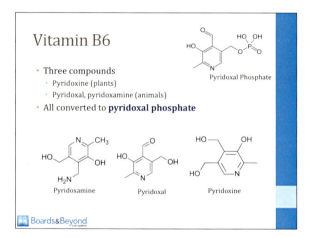

Pyridoxal phosphate
Vitamin B6

- Co-factor in many different reactions
- Aminotransferase reactions (**amino acids**)

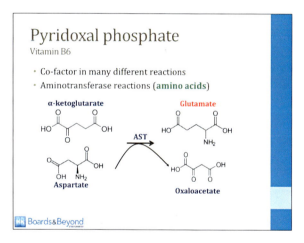

Pyridoxal phosphate
Neurotransmitters

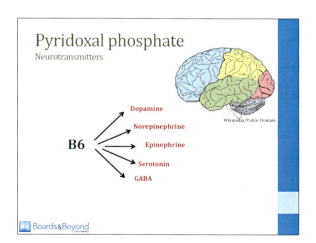

Cystathionine

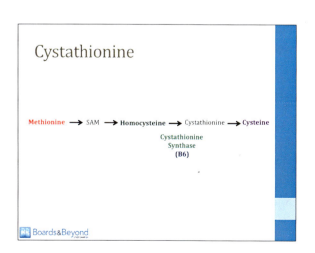

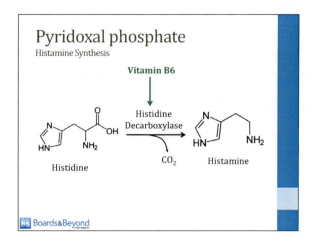
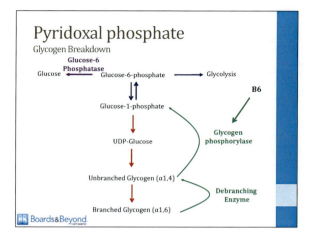
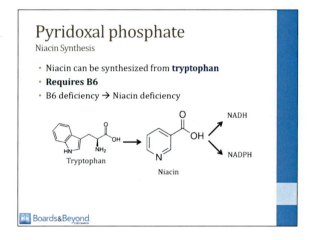
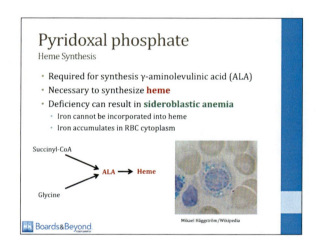
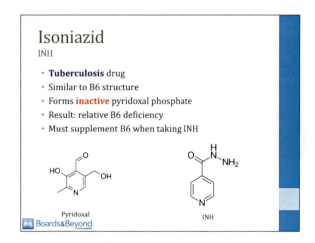
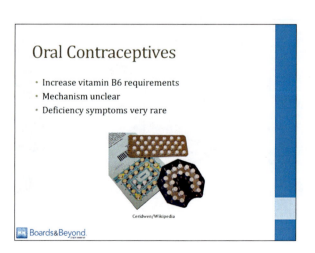

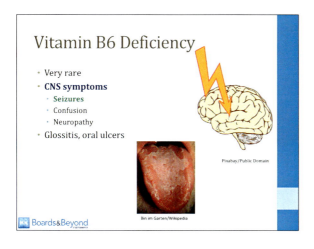
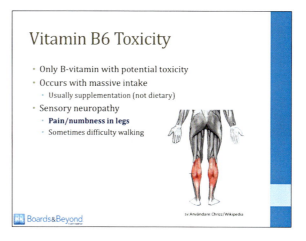
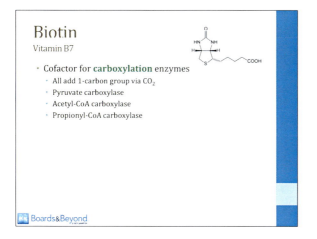
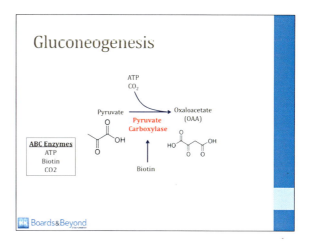
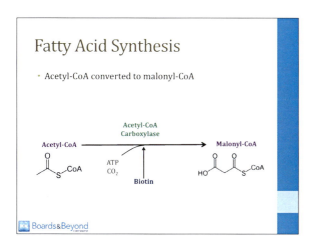
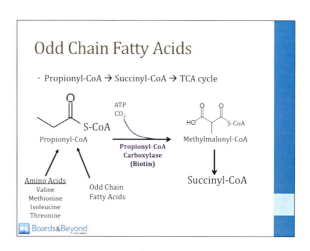

Biotin
Vitamin B7

- Deficiency
  - Very rare (vitamin widely distributed)
  - Massive consumption raw egg whites (avidin)
  - Dermatitis, glossitis, loss of appetite, nausea

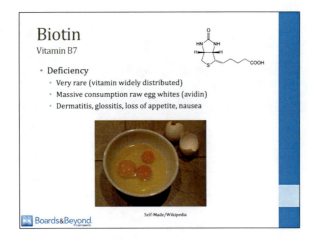

B Vitamins: Absorption

- All absorbed from diet in **small intestine**
- Most in **jejunum**
- Exception is B12: terminal ileum

Folate and Vitamin B12

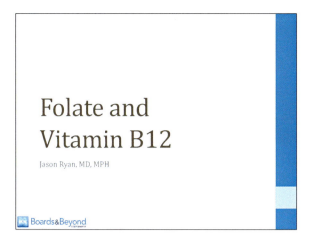

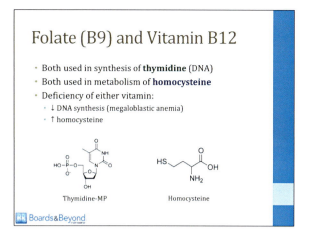

Folate (B9) and Vitamin B12

- Both used in synthesis of **thymidine** (DNA)
- Both used in metabolism of **homocysteine**
- Deficiency of either vitamin:
  - ↓ DNA synthesis (megaloblastic anemia)
  - ↑ homocysteine

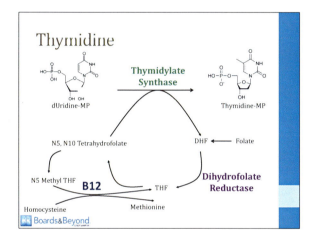

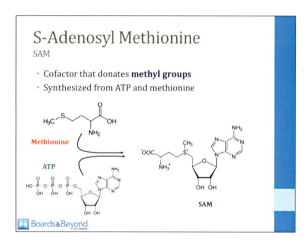

S-Adenosyl Methionine
SAM

- Cofactor that donates **methyl groups**
- Synthesized from ATP and methionine

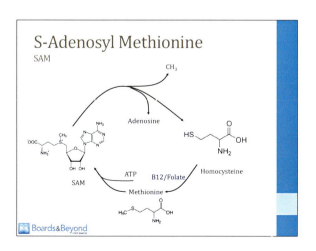

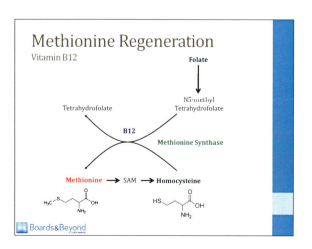

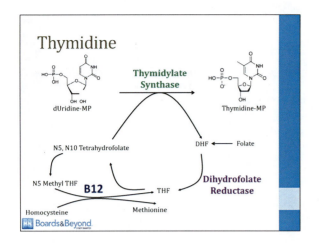
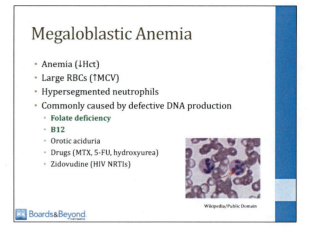
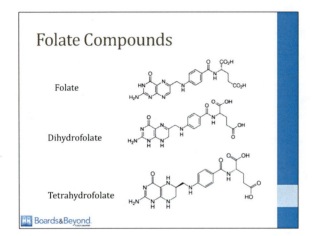
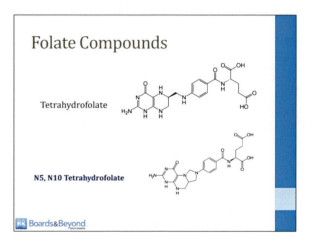
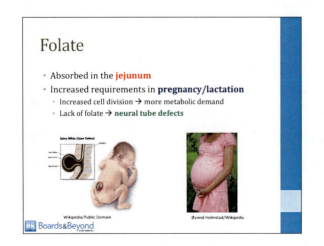
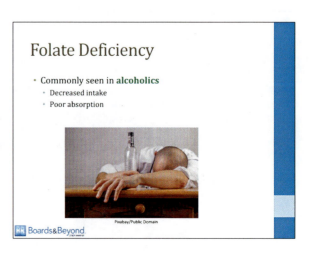

Folate Deficiency

- Poor absorption/utilization certain drugs
  - Phenytoin
  - Trimethoprim
  - Methotrexate

```
         Plasma | GI Tract
DHF ← Folate  ||  Folate
    ↘              ↑
  Dihydrofolate   Phenytoin
    Reductase
THF              Trimethoprim
                 Methotrexate
```

Cobalamin
Vitamin B12

- Large, complex structure (corrin ring)
- Contains element **cobalt**
- Only synthesized by bacteria
- Found in meats

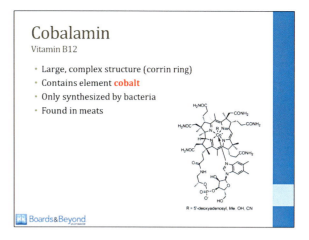

R = 5'-deoxyadenosyl, Me, OH, CN

Cobalamin
Vitamin B12

- One major role unique from folate
- **Odd chain fatty acid** metabolism
  - Conversion to succinyl CoA
  - Deficiency: ↑levels **methylmalonic acid**
  - Probably contributes to **peripheral neuropathy**
  - **Myelin** synthesis affected in B12 deficiency
  - Peripheral neuropathy not seen in folate deficiency

B12 Neuropathy

- Subacute combined degeneration (SCD)
- Involves **dorsal spinal columns**
- Defective **myelin** formation (unclear mechanism)
- Bilateral symptoms
- Legs >> arms
- Paresthesias
- Ataxia
- Loss of vibration and position sense
- Can progress: severe weakness, paraplegia

Odd Chain Fatty Acids
Vitamin B12

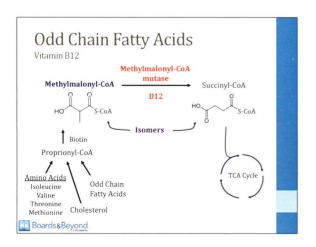

Odd Chain Fatty Acids
Vitamin B12

↑MMA: hallmark of B12 Deficiency
Not seen in folate deficiency

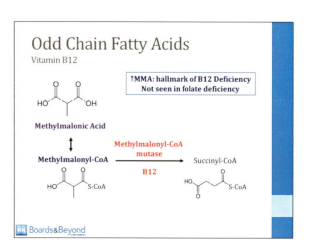

Cobalamin
Vitamin B12

- Liver stores **years** worth of vitamin B_{12}
- Deficiency from poor diet very rare

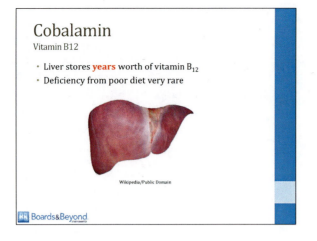

Pernicious Anemia

- Autoimmune destruction of **gastric parietal cells**
- Loss of secretion of **intrinsic factor**
- IF necessary for B12 absorption **terminal ileum**

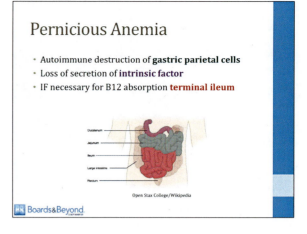

Pernicious Anemia

- Chronic inflammation of **gastric body**
- More common among **women**
- Complex immunology
  - Antibodies against parietal cells
  - Antibodies against intrinsic factor
  - **Type II hypersensitivity** features
  - Also autoreactive CD4 T-cells
- Associated with **HLA-DR antigens**
- Associated with **gastric adenocarcinoma**

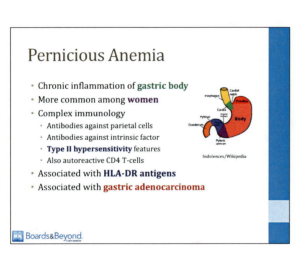

B12/Cobalamin
Other deficiency causes

- Ileum resection/dysfunction
  - Crohn's disease
- Loss of intrinsic factor from stomach
  - Gastric bypass
- **Diphyllobothrium latum**
  - Helminth (tapeworm)
  - Transmission from eating infected fish
  - Consumes B12

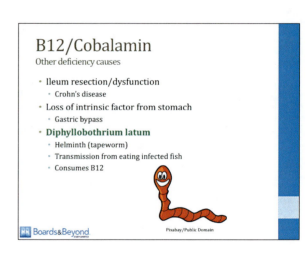

B12 Deficiency
Diagnosis

- Low serum B12
- High serum methylmalonic acid
- Antibodies to intrinsic factor (pernicious anemia)
- Schilling test
  - Classic diagnostic test for pernicious anemia
  - Oral radiolabeled B12
  - IM B12 to saturate liver receptors
  - Normal result: Radiolabeled B12 detectable to urine
  - Can repeat with oral IF

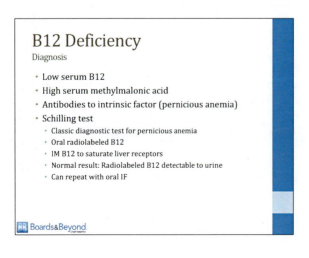

B12 Deficiency
Treatment

- Liquid injection available
- Often given SQ/IM
- Should see increase in reticulocytes

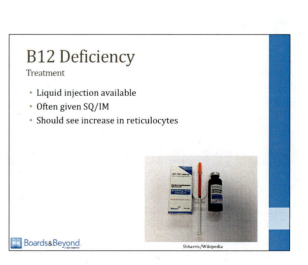

Anemia Classification

- MCV commonly used to classify anemias

Microcytic MCV<80	Normocytic MCV 80-100	Macrocytic MCV>100
Iron deficiency	Iron deficiency	Folate/B12 deficiency
Anemia Chronic Disease	Anemia Chronic Disease	Orotic Aciduria
Thalassemia	Hemolysis	Liver disease
Lead poisoning	Aplastic anemia	Alcoholism
Sideroblastic Anemia	Kidney disease	Reticulocytosis

Other Vitamins

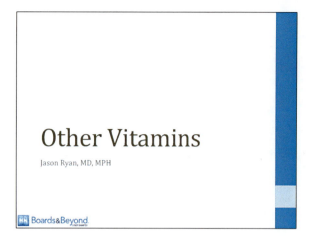

Other Vitamins
Jason Ryan, MD, MPH

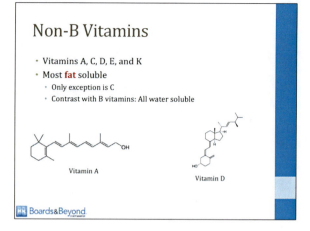

Non-B Vitamins
- Vitamins A, C, D, E, and K
- Most **fat** soluble
  - Only exception is C
  - Contrast with B vitamins: All water soluble

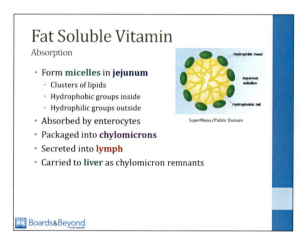

Fat Soluble Vitamin
Absorption
- Form **micelles** in **jejunum**
  - Clusters of lipids
  - Hydrophobic groups inside
  - Hydrophilic groups outside
- Absorbed by enterocytes
- Packaged into **chylomicrons**
- Secreted into **lymph**
- Carried to **liver** as chylomicron remnants

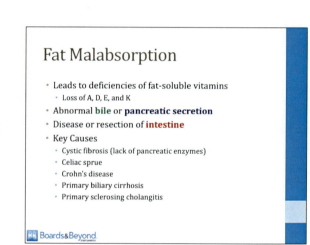

Fat Malabsorption
- Leads to deficiencies of fat-soluble vitamins
  - Loss of A, D, E, and K
- Abnormal **bile** or **pancreatic secretion**
- Disease or resection of **intestine**
- Key Causes
  - Cystic fibrosis (lack of pancreatic enzymes)
  - Celiac sprue
  - Crohn's disease
  - Primary biliary cirrhosis
  - Primary sclerosing cholangitis

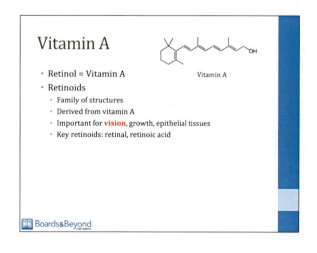

Vitamin A
- Retinol = Vitamin A
- Retinoids
  - Family of structures
  - Derived from vitamin A
  - Important for **vision**, growth, epithelial tissues
  - Key retinoids: retinal, retinoic acid

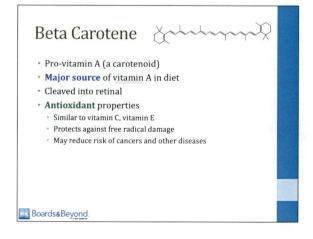

Beta Carotene
- Pro-vitamin A (a carotenoid)
- **Major source** of vitamin A in diet
- Cleaved into retinal
- **Antioxidant** properties
  - Similar to vitamin C, vitamin E
  - Protects against free radical damage
  - May reduce risk of cancers and other diseases

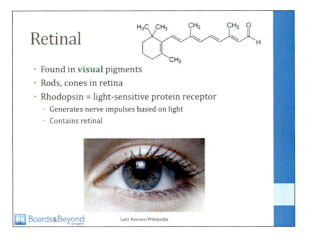
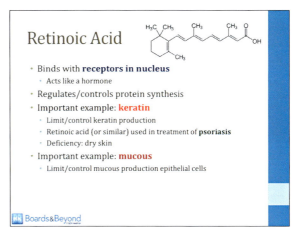
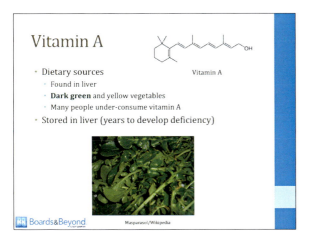
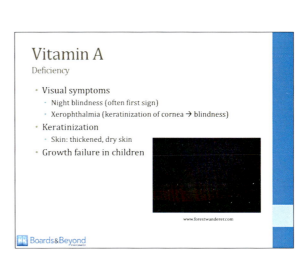
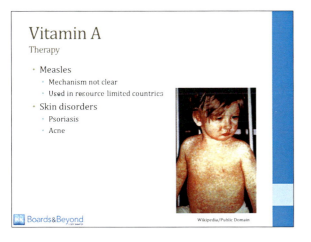
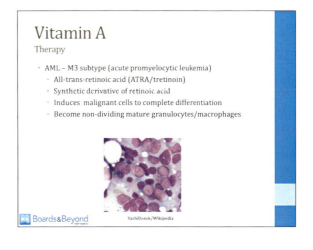

Vitamin A
Excess

- Hypervitaminosis A
- Usually from chronic, excessive supplements
- Dry, itchy skin
- Enlarged liver

Isotretinoin
Accutane

- 13-*cis*-retinoic acid
- Effective for **acne**
- Highly teratogenic
- OCP and/or pregnancy test prior to Rx

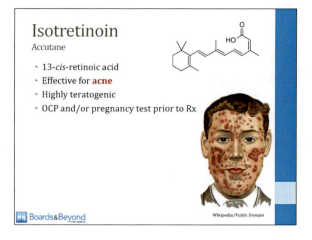

Vitamin C
Ascorbic Acid

- Only water-soluble non-B vitamin
- **Antioxidant** properties
- Found in fruits and vegetables
- Three key roles:
  - Absorption of iron
  - Collagen synthesis
  - Dopamine synthesis

Iron Absorption

- Heme iron
  - Found in meats
  - Easily absorbed
- Non-heme iron
  - Absorbed in Fe^{2+} state
  - Aided by vitamin C
  - Important for vegans
- Methemoglobinemia
  - Fe^{3+} iron in heme
  - Rx: Vitamin C

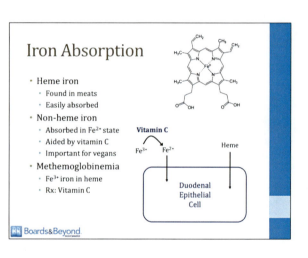

Collagen Synthesis

- Post-translational modification of collagen
- Hydroxylation of specific **proline and lysine** residues
- Occurs in **endoplasmic reticulum**
- Deficiency → ↓ collagen → scurvy

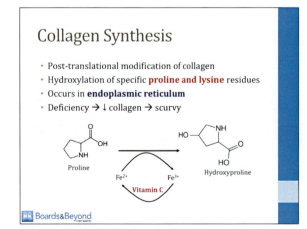

Tyrosine Metabolism

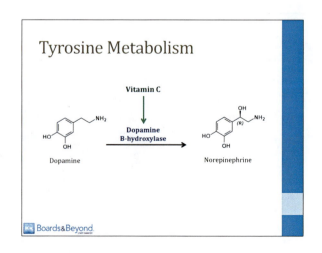

Scurvy

- Vitamin C deficiency syndrome
- Defective **collagen** synthesis
- Sore gums, loose teeth
- Fragile blood vessels → easy bruising
- Historical disorder
  - Common on long sea voyages
  - Sailors ate limes to prevent scurvy ("Limey")
- Seen with "**tea and toast**" diet (no fruits/vegetables)

Vitamin C Excess

- Nausea, vomiting, diarrhea
- **Iron overload**
  - Predisposed patients
  - Frequent transfusions, hemochromatosis
- **Kidney stones**
  - Calcium oxalate stones
  - Vitamin C can be metabolized into oxalate

Smoking

- Increased vitamin C requirements
- Likely due to antioxidant properties
- Deficient levels common
- Scurvy or definite symptoms rare

Vitamin D

- Vitamin D_2 is ergocalciferol
  - Found in plants
- Vitamin D_3 is cholecalciferol
  - Found in fortified milk
- Two sources D_3:
  - Diet
  - **Sunlight** (skin synthesizes D_3)

Vitamin D Activation

- Vitamin D_3 from sun/food inert
  - No biologic activity
- Must be **hydroxylated** to become active
- Step 1: 25 hydroxylation
  - Occurs in **liver**
  - Constant activity
- Step 2: 1 hydroxylation
  - Occurs in **kidney**
  - Regulated by PTH

Vitamin D Activation

- Liver: Converts to 25-OH Vitamin D (calcidiol)
- Kidney: Converts to 1,25-OH_2 Vitamin D (**calcitriol**)
- 1,25-OH_2 Vitamin D = active form

Vitamin D Activation

- 25-OH Vitamin D = **storage form**
  - Constantly produced by liver
  - Available for activation by kidney as needed
- Serum [25-OH VitD] best indicator vitamin D status
  - Long half-life
  - Liver production not regulated

Vitamin D and the Kidney

- **Proximal tubule** converts vitamin D to active form
- Can occur independent of kidney in **sarcoidosis**
  - Leads to hypercalcemia

$$25\text{-OH Vitamin D} \xrightarrow{1\alpha\text{ - hydroxylase}} 1,25\text{-OH}_2 \text{ Vitamin D}$$

(PTH + stimulates 1α-hydroxylase)

Vitamin D Function

- GI: ↑Ca^{2+} and PO_4^{3-} absorption
  - **Major mechanism of clinical effects**
  - Raises Ca, increases bone mineralization
- Bone: ↑Ca^{2+} and PO_4^{3-} resorption
  - Process of demineralizing bones
  - Paradoxical effect
  - Occurs at abnormally high levels

Suda T et al. Bone effects of vitamin D - Discrepancies between in vivo and in vitro studies
Arch Biochem Biophys. 2012 Jul 1;523(1):22-9

Vitamin D Deficiency

- Poor GI absorption Ca^{2+} and PO_4^{3-}
  - Hypophosphatemia
  - **Hypocalcemia** (tetany, seizures)
- Bone: **poor mineralization**
  - Adults: Osteomalacia
  - Children: Rickets

Osteomalacia

- Children and adults
- Occurs in areas of bone turnover
  - Bone remodeling constantly occurring
  - Osteoclasts clear bone
  - Osteoblasts lay down new bone ("osteoid")
- ↓ Vitamin D = ↓ mineralization of newly formed bone
- Clinical features
  - **Bone pain**/tenderness
  - Fractures
- PTH levels very high
- CXR: Reduced bone density

Rickets

- Only occurs in **children**
- Deficient mineralization of growth plate
- **Growth plate** processes
  - Chondrocytes hypertrophy/proliferate
  - Vascular invasion → mineralization
- ↓ Vitamin D:
  - Growth plate thickens without mineralization
- Clinical features
  - Bone pain
  - Distal forearm/knee most affected (rapid growth)
  - Delayed closure fontanelles
  - **Bowing** of femur/tibia (classic X-ray finding)

Rickets

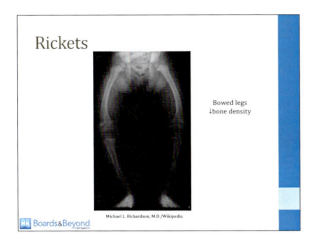

Bowed legs
↓bone density

Vitamin D in Renal Failure

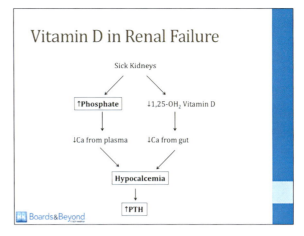

Vitamin D
Sources

- Natural sources:
  - Oily fish (salmon)
  - Liver
  - Egg yolk
- Most milk **fortified** with vitamin D
- Rickets largely eliminated due to fortification

Vitamin D
Breast Feeding

- Breast milk low in vitamin D
  - Even if mother has sufficient levels
- Lower in women with **dark skin**
- Most infants get little sun exposure
- Exclusively breast fed infants → supplementation

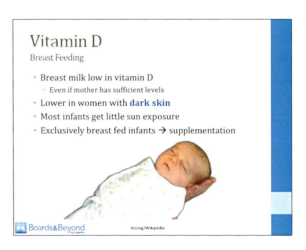

Vitamin D
Excess

- Hypervitaminosis D
  - Massive consumption calcitriol supplements
  - **Sarcoidosis**
  - Granulomatous macrophages express 1α-hydroxylase
- Hypercalcemia, hypercalciuria
- Kidney stones
- Confusion

Vitamin E
Tocopherol

- Antioxidant
- Key role in protecting **RBCs** from oxidative damage

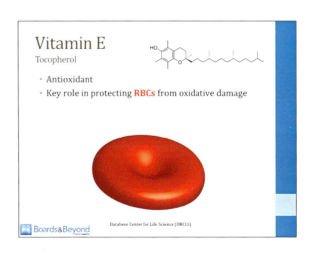

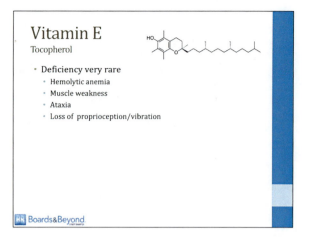
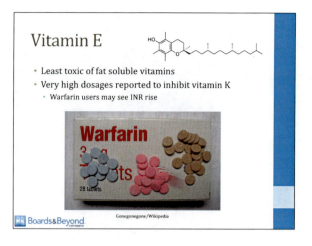
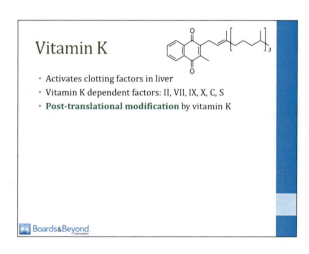
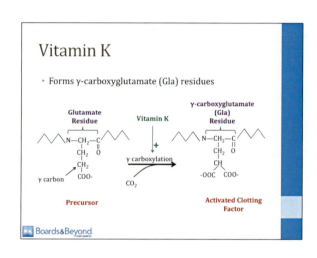
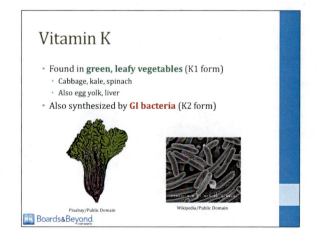
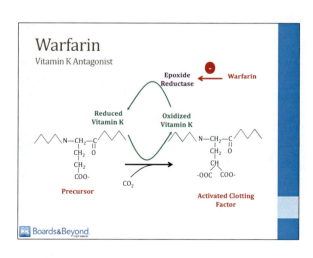

Vitamin K Deficiency

- Results in **bleeding** ("coagulopathy")
- Deficiency of vitamin K-dependent factors
- Key lab findings:
  - **Elevated PT/INR**
  - Can see elevated PTT (less sensitive)
  - Normal bleeding time
- Dietary deficiency rare
- GI bacteria produce sufficient quantities

Vitamin K Deficiency
Causes

- Warfarin therapy (deficient action)
- **Antibiotics**
  - Decrease GI bacteria
  - May alter warfarin dose requirement
- **Newborn babies**
  - Sterile GI tract at birth
  - Insufficient vitamin K in breast milk
  - Risk of neonatal hemorrhage
  - Babies given IM vitamin K at birth

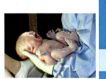

Zinc

- Cofactor for many (100+) enzymes
- Deficiency in children
  - Poor growth
  - Impaired **sexual development**
- Deficiency in children/adults
  - Poor **wound healing**
  - Loss of **taste** (required by taste buds)
  - Immune dysfunction (required for cytokine production)
  - Dermatitis: red skin, pustules (patients on TPN)

Zinc

- Found in meat, chicken
- Absorbed mostly in duodenum (similar to iron)
- Risk factors for deficiency
  - Alcoholism (low zinc associated with cirrhosis)
  - Chronic renal disease
  - Malabsorption

Acrodermatitis enteropathica

- Rare, autosomal recessive disease
- Zinc absorption impaired
- Mutations in gene for zinc transportation
- Dermatitis
  - Hyperpigmented (often red) skin
  - Classically perioral and perianal
  - Also in arms/legs
- Other symptoms
  - Loss of hair, diarrhea, poor growth
  - Immune dysfunction (recurrent infections)

Zinc fingers

- Protein segments that contain zinc
  - "Domain," "Motif"
- Found in proteins that bind proteins, RNA, DNA
- Often bind specific DNA sequences
- Influence/modify genes and gene activity

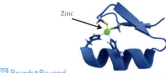

Lipid Metabolism

Lipid Metabolism
Jason Ryan, MD, MPH

Lipids
- Mostly carbon and hydrogen
- Not soluble in water
- Many types:
  - Fatty acids
  - Triglycerides
  - Cholesterol
  - Phospholipids
  - Steroids
  - Glycolipids

Lipids

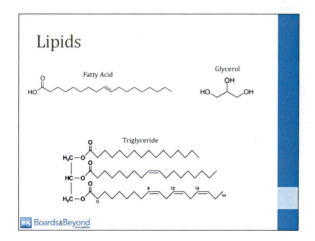

Lipids

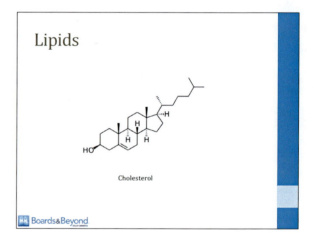

Cholesterol

Lipoproteins
Particles of lipids and proteins

- Chylomicrons
- Very low-density lipoprotein (VLDL)
- Intermediate-density lipoprotein (IDL)
- Low density lipoproteins (LDL)
- High-density lipoprotein (HDL)

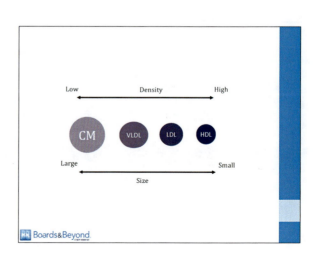

Apolipoproteins

- Proteins that bind lipids
- Found in lipoproteins
- Various functions:
  - Surface receptors
  - Co-factors for enzymes

Absorption of Fatty Acids

- Fatty acids → Triglycerides
- Packaged into **chylomicrons** by intestinal cells
- To lymph → blood stream

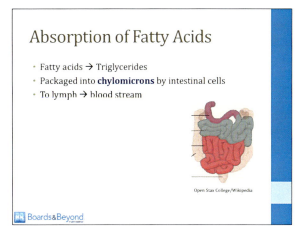

Absorption of Cholesterol

- **Cholesteryl esters** formed in enterocytes
- Acyl-CoA cholesterol acyltransferase (**ACAT**)
- Packaged into chylomicrons by intestinal cells
- To lymph → blood stream

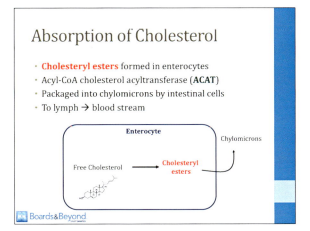

Cholesteryl Esters

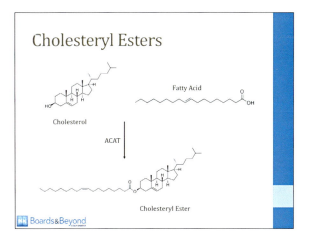

Chylomicrons

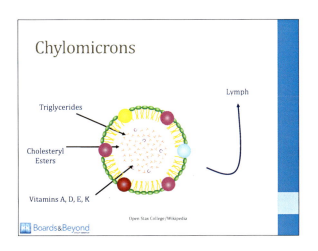

Apolipoprotein B48

- Found only on chylomicrons
- Contains 48% of apo-B protein
- Required for **secretion from enterocytes**

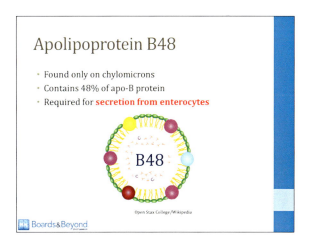

Lipoprotein Lipase
LPL

- **Extracellular** enzyme
- Anchored to **capillary walls**
- Mostly found in adipose tissue, muscle, and heart
  - Not in liver → liver has hepatic lipase
- Converts triglycerides → fatty acids (and glycerol)
- Fatty acids used for storage (adipose) or fuel
- Requires **apo C-II** for activation

Other Apolipoproteins

- **C-II**
  - Co-factor for lipoprotein lipase
  - Carried by: Chylomicrons, VLDL/IDL
- **Apo E**
  - Binds to liver receptors
  - Required for uptake of remnants
- Both from **HDL**

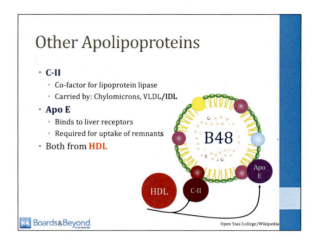

Chylomicrons

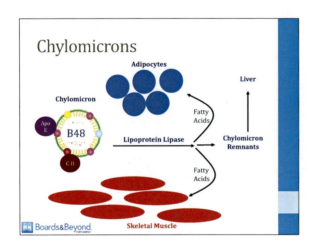

Chylomicron Remnants

- Apo-E receptors on **liver**
- Take up remnants via receptor-mediated endocytosis
- Usually only present after meals (clear 1-5hrs)
- Milky appearance

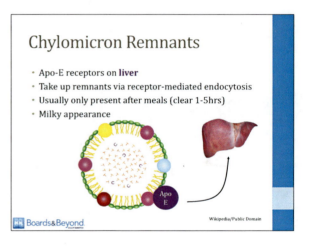

Chylomicrons
Summary

- Secreted from enterocytes with Apo48
- Pick up Apo C-II and ApoE from HDL
- Carry triglycerides and cholesteryl esters
- Deliver triglycerides to cells
  - Lipoprotein lipase stimulates (C-II co-factor) breakdown
- Return to liver as chylomicron remnants
  - ApoE receptors on liver

Cholesterol Synthesis

- Only the liver can synthesize cholesterol

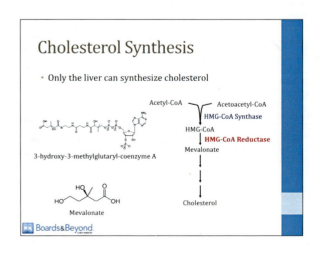

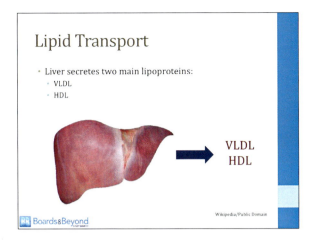
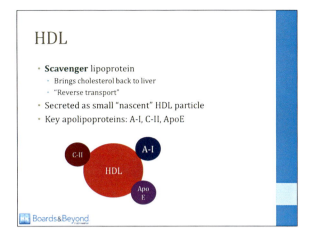
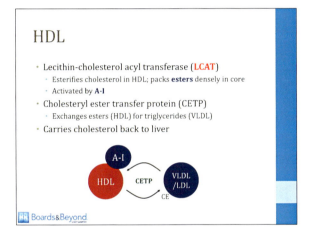
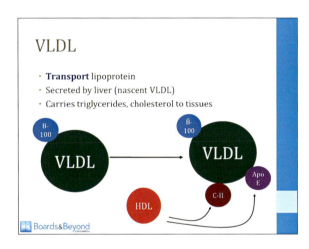
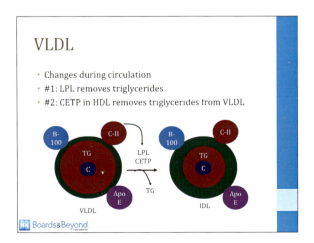
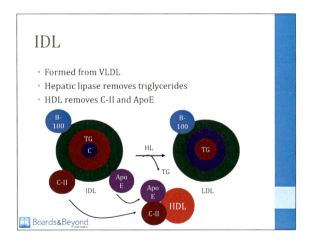

Hepatic Lipase

- Found in **liver** capillaries
- Similar function to LPL (releases fatty acids)
- Very important for IDL → LDL conversion
- Absence HL → absence IDL/LDL conversion

LDL

- Small amount of triglycerides
- High concentration of cholesterol/cholesteryl esters
- Transfers cholesterol to cells with **LDL receptor**
  - Receptor-mediated endocytosis
- LDL receptors recognize B100

Foam Cells

- **Macrophages** filled with cholesterol
- Found in atherosclerotic plaques
- Contain LDL receptors and LDL

Summary

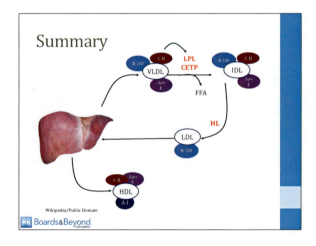

Lipoprotein Composition

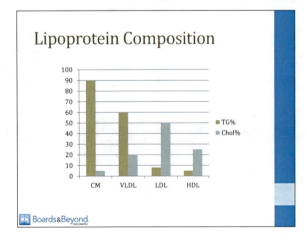

Lipoprotein(a)
Lp(a)

- Modified form of LDL
- Contains large glycoprotein apolipoprotein(a)
- Elevated levels risk factor for cardiovascular disease
- Not routinely measured
- No proven therapy for high levels

Abetalipoproteinemia

- Autosomal recessive disorder
- Defect in MTP
  - Microsomal triglyceride transfer protein
- MTP forms/secretes lipoproteins with apo-B
  - Chylomicrons from intestine (B48)
  - VLDL from liver (B100)

Abetalipoproteinemia
Clinical Features

- Presents in infancy
  - Steatorrhea
  - Abdominal distension
  - Failure to thrive
- Fat-soluble vitamin deficiencies
  - Especially vitamin E (ataxia, weakness, hemolysis)
  - Vitamin A (poor vision)
- Lipid accumulation in enterocytes on biopsy

Abetalipoproteinemia
Lab Findings

- Low or zero VLDL/IDL/LDL
- Very low triglyceride and total cholesterol levels
- Low vitamin E levels
- Acanthocytosis
  - Abnormal RBC membrane lipids

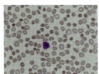

Rola Zamel, Razi Khan,
Rebecca L Pollex and Robert A Hegele

Hyperlipidemia

Hyperlipidemia
Jason Ryan, MD, MPH

Lipid Measurements
- Total Cholesterol
- LDL-C
- HDL-C
- TG

Friedewald Formula

$$LDL\text{-}C = \text{Total Chol} - HDL\text{-}C - \frac{TG}{5}$$

Hyperlipidemia
- Elevated total cholesterol, LDL, or triglycerides
- Risk factor for coronary disease and stroke
- Modifiable – often related to lifestyle factors
  - Sedentary lifestyle
  - Saturated and trans-fatty acid foods
  - Lack of fiber

Secondary Hyperlipidemia

Selected Causes of Hyperlipidemia
Nephrotic syndrome (LDL)
Alcohol use (TG)
Pregnancy (TG)
Beta blockers (TG)
HCTZ (TC, LDL, TG)

Signs of Hyperlipidemia
- Most patients have no signs/symptoms
- Physical findings occur in patients with severe ↑lipids
- Usually familial syndrome

Signs of Hyperlipidemia
- Xanthomas
  - Plaques of lipid-laden histiocytes
  - Appear as skin bumps or on eyelids
- Tendinous Xanthoma
  - Lipid deposits in tendons
  - Common in Achilles
- Corneal arcus
  - Lipid deposit in cornea
  - Seen on fundoscopy

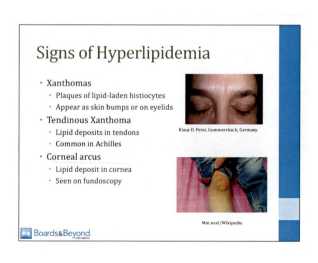

Klaus D. Peter, Gummersbach, Germany

Min.neel/Wikipedia

Pancreatitis

- Elevated triglycerides (>1000) → acute pancreatitis
- Exact mechanism unclear
- May involve increased **chylomicrons** in plasma
  - Chylomicrons usually formed after meals and cleared
  - Always present when triglycerides > 1000mg/dL
  - May obstruct capillaries → ischemia
  - Vessel damage can expose triglycerides to pancreatic lipases
  - Triglycerides breakdown → **free fatty acids**
  - Acid → tissue injury → pancreatitis

Familial Dyslipidemias

- Type I – **Hyperchylomicronemia**
- Autosomal recessive
- ↑↑↑TG (>1000; milky plasma appearance)
- ↑↑↑ chylomicrons

Familial Dyslipidemias

- Type I – **Hyperchylomicronemia**
- Severe LPL dysfunction
  - LPL deficient
  - LPL co-factor deficient (apolipoprotein C-II)
- Recurrent pancreatitis
- Enlarged liver, xanthomas
- Treatment: Very low fat diet
  - Reports of normal lifespan
  - No apparent ↑risk atherosclerosis

Familial Dyslipidemias

- Type II – **Familial Hypercholesterolemia**
  - Autosomal **dominant**
  - Few or zero LDL receptors
  - **Very high LDL** (>300 heterozygote; >700 homozygote)
  - Tendon xanthomas, corneal arcus
  - **Severe atherosclerosis** (can have MI in 20s)

Familial Dyslipidemias

- Type III – **Familial Dysbetalipoproteinemia**
  - Apo-E2 subtype of Apo-E
  - Poorly cleared by liver
  - Accumulation of chylomicron remnants and VLDL
    - (collectively know as β-lipoproteins)
  - Elevated total cholesterol and triglycerides
  - Usually mild (TC>300 mg/dl)
  - Xanthomas
  - **Premature coronary disease**

ApoE and Alzheimer's

- ApoE2
  - Decreased risk of Alzheimer's
- ApoE4
  - Increased risk of Alzheimer's

Familial Dyslipidemias

- Type IV **Hypertriglyceridemia**
  - Autosomal **dominant**
  - VLDL overproduction or impaired catabolism
  - ↑**TG (200-500)**
  - ↑VLDL
  - Associated with diabetes type II
  - Often diagnosed on routine screening bloodwork
  - Increased coronary risk/premature coronary disease

Lipid Drugs

Lipid Drugs
Jason Ryan, MD, MPH

The "Cholesterol Panel"
"Lipid Panel"
- Total Cholesterol
- LDL-C
- HDL-C
- TG

Friedewald Formula

$$LDL\text{-}C = TotChol - HDL\text{-}C - \frac{TG}{5}$$

LDL Cholesterol
- "Bad" cholesterol
- Associated with CV risk
- <100 mg/dl very good
- >200 mg/dl high
- Evidence that treating high levels reduces risk

HDL Cholesterol
- "Good" cholesterol
- Inversely associated with risk
- <45mg/dl low
- Little evidence that raising low levels reduces risk

Trigylcerides
- Normal TG level <150mg/dl
- Levels > 1000 can cause **pancreatitis**
- Elevated TG levels modestly associated with CAD
- Little evidence that lowering high levels reduces risk

Pancreatitis
- Elevated triglycerides → acute pancreatitis
- Exact mechanism unclear
- May involve increased **chylomicrons** in plasma
  - Chylomicrons usually formed after meals and cleared
  - Always present when triglycerides > 1000mg/dL
  - May obstruct capillaries → ischemia
  - Vessel damage can expose triglycerides to pancreatic lipases
  - Triglycerides breakdown → free fatty acids
  - Acid → tissue injury → pancreatitis

Treating Hyperlipidemia

- Usually treat **elevated LDL-C with statins**
- Rarely treat elevated TG or low HDL-C
- Secondary prevention
  - Patients with coronary or vascular disease
  - Strong evidence that lipid lowering drugs benefit
- Primary prevention
  - Not all patients benefit the same
  - Benefit depends on risk of CV disease

Guidelines
Lipid Drug Therapy

- Old Cholesterol Guidelines set LDL-C goal
  - Diabetes or CAD: Goal LDL <100
  - 2 or more risk factors: Goal LDL <130
  - 0 or 1 risk factor: Goal LDL <160
- New guidelines require risk calculator
  - Treat patients if risk above limit (usually 5%/year)
  - No LDL goal
- **Statins 1st line** majority of hyperlipidemia patients

Treating TG or HDL

- Rarely treat for TG or HDL alone
- Many LDL drugs improve TG/HDL
- Few data showing a benefit of treatment

Treating TG or HDL

- Triglycerides
  - >500
  - High Non-HDL cholesterol (TC – HDL)
- Low HDL
  - Patients with established CAD

Lipid Lowering Drugs

- Statins
- Niacin
- Fibrates
- Absorption blockers
- Bile acid resins
- Omega-3 fatty acids

Diet/exercise/weight loss = GREAT way to reduce cholesterol levels and CV risk

Statins
Lovastatin, Atorvastatin, Simvastatin

- Act on liver synthesis
- HMG-CoA reductase inhibitors
- ↓cholesterol synthesis in liver
- **↑LDL receptors in liver**
- Major effect: ↓ LDL decrease
- Some ↓TG, ↑HDL
- **Excellent outcomes data** (↓MI/Death)
- ↑LFTs

3-hydroxy-3-methylglutaryl-coenzyme A
HMG-CoA

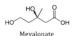

HMG-CoA Reductase

Mevalonate

Statin Muscle Problems

- Many muscle symptoms associated with statins
- Mechanism poorly understood
- Low levels of **coenzyme** Q in muscles
- Many patients take CoQ 10 supplements
- Theoretical benefit for muscle aches on statins

Statin Muscle Problems

- Myalgias
  - Weakness, soreness
  - Normal CK levels
- Myositis
  - Like myalgias, increased CK
- Rhabdomyolysis
  - Weakness, muscle pain, dark urine
  - CKs in 1000s
  - Acute renal failure → death
  - ↑risk with some drugs (cyclosporine, gemfibrozil)

Hydrophilic vs. Lipophilic
Statins

- Hydrophilic statins
  - Pravastatin, fluvastatin, **rosuvastatin**
  - May cause less myalgias
- Lipophilic statins
  - **Atorvastatin**, simvastatin, lovastatin

P450

- Statins metabolized by liver P450 system
- Interactions with other drugs
- Inhibitors increase ↑ risk LFTs/myalgias
  - i.e. grapefruit juice

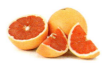

Citrus_paradisi/Wikipedia

Niacin

- Complex, incompletely understood mechanism
- Overall effect: LDL ↓↓ **HDL ↑↑**
- Often used when HDL is low

Niacin

↓FA mobilization → ↓TG

↓VLDL → ↓LDL

↓HDL breakdown → ↑HDL

Niacin

- Major side effects is **flushing**
  - Stimulates release of prostaglandins in skin
  - **Face** turns red, warm
  - Can blunt with **aspirin** (inhibits prostaglandin) prior to Niacin
  - Fades with time

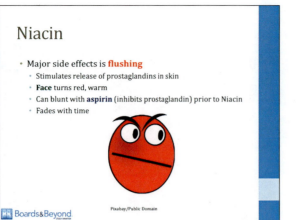

Niacin

- Hyperglycemia
  - Insulin resistance (mechanism incompletely understood)
  - Avoid in diabetes
- Hyperuricemia

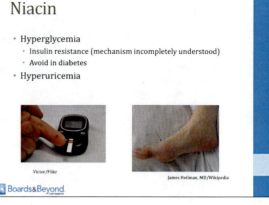

Fibrates
Gemfibrozil, clofibrate, bezafibrate, fenofibrate

- Activate **PPAR-a**
  - Modifies gene transcription
  - ↑ activity lipoprotein lipase
  - ↑ liver fatty acid oxidation → ↓ VLDL
- Major overall effect → TG breakdown
- Used for patients with very **high triglycerides**

Fibrates
Gemfibrozil, clofibrate, bezafibrate, fenofibrate

- Side effects
  - ↑ LFTs
  - Cholesterol gallstones
  - Myositis
- Gemfibrozil: rhabdomyolysis with statins
  - Inhibits cytochrome P450 enzymes
  - Increases statin levels in plasma
  - Increased likelihood of rhabdomyolysis
  - Only fenofibrate given with statins

Absorption blockers
Ezetimibe

- Blocks cholesterol absorption
- Works at **intestinal brush border**
- Blocks dietary **cholesterol** absorption
  - Highly selective for cholesterol
  - Does not affect fat-soluble vitamins, triglycerides

Absorption blockers
Ezetimibe

- Result: ↑LDL receptors on liver
- Modest reduction LDL
- Some ↓TG, ↑HDL
- Weak data on hard outcomes (MI, death)
- ↑LFTs
- Diarrhea

Bile Acid Resins
Cholestyramine, colestipol, colesevelam

- Old drugs; rarely used
- Prevent intestinal reabsorption bile
  - Cholesterol → bile → GI tract → reabsorption
- Resins lead to more bile excretion in stool
- Liver converts cholesterol → bile to makeup losses
- Modest lowering LDL
- Miserable for patients: **Bloating, bad taste**
- Can't absorb certain fat soluble vitamins
- Cholesterol gallstones

Omega-3 Fatty Acids

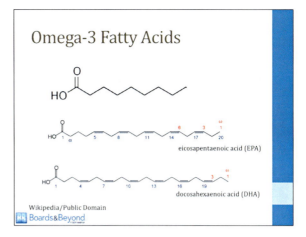

Wikipedia/Public Domain

Omega-3 Fatty Acids

- Found in fish oil
- Consumption associated with ↓CV events
- Incorporated into cell membranes
- **Reduce VLDL production**
- **Lowers triglycerides** (~25 to 30%)
- Modest ↑ HDL
- Commercial supplements available (Lovaza)
- GI side effects: nausea, diarrhea, "fishy" taste

PCSK9 Inhibitors
Alirocumab, Evolocumab

- FDA approval in 2015
- PCSK9 → **degradation of LDL receptors**
  - Binds to LDL receptor
  - LDL receptor transported to lysosome
- Alirocumab/Evolocumab: Antibodies
- Inactivate PCSK9
  - ↓ LDL-receptor degradation
  - ↑ LDL receptors on hepatocytes
  - ↓ LDL cholesterol in plasma

PCSK9 Inhibitors
Alirocumab, Evolocumab

- Given by subcutaneous injection
- Results in significant LDL reductions (>60%)
- Major adverse effect is injection site skin reaction
- Some association with memory problems

Lysosomal Storage Diseases

Lysosomal Storage Diseases

Jason Ryan, MD, MPH

Lysosomes

- Membrane-bound organelles of cells
- Contain enzymes
- Breakdown numerous biological structures
  - Proteins, nucleic acids, carbohydrates, lipids
- Digest obsolete components of the cell

Mediran/Wikipedia

Lysosomal Storage Diseases

- Absence of lysosomal enzyme
- Inability to breakdown complex molecules
- Accumulation → disease
- Most autosomal recessive
- Most have no treatment or cure

Sphingolipids

- **Sphingosine**: long chain "amino alcohol"
- Addition of **fatty acid** to NH2 = **Ceramide**

Sphingosine

Ceramide

Ceramide Derivatives

- Modification of "head group" on ceramide
- Yields glycosphingolipids, sulfatides, others
- Very important structures for **nerve tissue**
- Lack of breakdown → accumulation **liver**, **spleen**

Head Group

Ceramide

Ceramide Trihexoside
Globotriaosylceramide (Gb3)

- Three sugar head group on ceramide
- Broken down by **α-galactosidase A**
- **Fabry's Disease**
  - Deficiency of α-galactosidase A
  - Accumulation of ceramide trihexoside

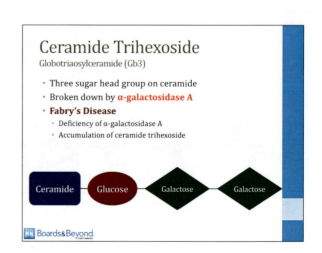

Ceramide — Glucose — Galactose — Galactose

Fabry's Disease

- **X-linked recessive** disease
- Slowly progressive symptoms
- Begins child → early adulthood

Fabry's Disease

- Neuropathy
  - Classically pain in limbs, **hands, feet**
- Skin: **angiokeratomas**
  - Small dark, red to purple raised spots
  - Dilated surface capillaries
- **Decreased sweat**

Fabry's Disease

- Renal disease
  - Proteinuria, renal failure
- Cardiac disease
  - Left ventricular hypertrophy
  - Heart failure

Fabry's Disease

- CNS problems
  - TIA/Stroke (early age)

Fabry's Disease

- Often misdiagnosed initially
- Enzyme replacement therapy available
  - Recombinant galactosidase

Fabry's Disease

- Classic case
  - Child with pain in hands/feet
  - Lack of sweat
  - Skin findings

Deficiency of α-galactosidase A
Accumulation of ceramide trihexoside

Glucocerebroside

- Glucose head group on ceramide
- Broken down by **glucocerebrosidase**
- **Gaucher's disease**
  - Deficiency of glucocerebrosidase
  - Accumulation of glucocerebroside

Gaucher's Disease

- Most common lysosomal storage disease
- Autosomal recessive
- More common among **Ashkenazi Jewish** population
- Lipids accumulate in spleen, liver, bones

Gaucher's Disease

- Hepatosplenomegaly:
  - **Splenomegaly**: most common initial sign
- Bones
  - Marrow: Anemia, thrombocytopenia, rarely leukopenia
  - Often **easy bruising** from low platelets
  - Avascular necrosis of joints (joint collapse)
- CNS (rare, neuropathic forms of disease)
  - Gaze palsy
  - Dementia
  - Ataxia

Gaucher's Disease

Gaucher Cell: *Macrophage* filled with lipid
"Crinkled paper"

Bone Crises

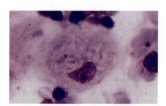

- Severe bone pain
- Due to bone infarction (ischemia)
- Infiltration of Gaucher cells in intramedullary space
- Intense pain, often with fever (like sickle cell)

Gaucher's Disease

- Type I
  - Most common form
  - Presents childhood to adult
  - Minimal CNS dysfunction
  - Hepatosplenomegaly, bruising, anemia, joint problems
  - Normal lifespan possible
  - Enzyme replacement therapy
  - Synthetic (recombinant DNA) glucocerebrosidase

Gaucher's Disease

- Type II
  - Presents in infancy with marked CNS symptoms
  - Death <2yrs
- Type III
  - Childhood onset; progressive dementia; shortened lifespan

Gaucher's Disease

- Classic case:
  - Child of Ashkenazi Jewish descent
  - Splenomegaly on exam
  - Anemia
  - Bruising (low platelets)
  - Joint pain/fractures

Deficiency of glucocerebrosidase
Accumulation of glucocerebroside

Sphingomyelin

- Phosphate-nitrogen head group
- Broken down by **sphingomyelinase**
- **Niemann-Pick disease**
- Deficiency of acid sphingomyelinase (ASM)
  - Accumulation of sphingomyelin

Niemann-Pick Disease

- Autosomal recessive
- More common among **Ashkenazi Jewish** population
- Splenomegaly, neurologic deficits
- Multiple subtypes of disease
- Presents in infancy to adulthood based on type

Niemann-Pick Disease

- **Hepatosplenomegaly**
  - 2° thrombocytopenia
- Progressive neuro impairment
  - Weakness: will worsen over time
  - Classic presentation: child that **loses motor skills**
- Pathology
  - Large macrophages with lipids
  - "**Foam cells**"
  - Spleen, bone marrow
- Severe forms: death <3-4yrs

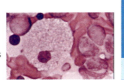

Cherry Red Spot

- Seen in many conditions:
  - Niemann-Pick
  - Tay-Sachs
  - Central retinal artery occlusion

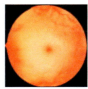

Jonathan Trobe, M.D./Wikipedia

Niemann-Pick Disease

- Classic case:
  - Previously well, healthy child
  - Weakness, loss of motor skills
  - Enlarged liver or spleen on physical exam
  - Cherry red spot

Deficiency of sphingomyelinase
Accumulation of sphingomyelin

Galactocerebroside

- Galactose head group
- Broken down by **galactocerebrosidase**
- Major component of **myelin**
- **Krabbe's Disease**
  - Deficiency of galactocerebrosidase
  - Abnormal metabolism of galactocerebroside

Krabbe's Disease

- Autosomal Recessive
- Usually presents <6 months of age
- Only neuro symptoms
- **Progressive weakness**
  - Developmental delay
  - Eventually floppy limbs, loss of head control
- Absent reflexes
- Optic atrophy: vision loss
- Often fever without infection
- Usually death <2 years

Globoid Cells

- Krabbe: globoid cell leukodystrophy
- Globoid cells in neuronal tissue
  - Globe-shaped cells
  - Often more than one nucleus

Gangliosides

- Contain head group with NANA
  - N-acetylneuraminic acid (also called sialic acid)
- Names GM1, GM2, GM3
  - G-ganglioside
  - M= # of NANA's (m=mono)
  - 1,2,3= Sugar sequence

Tay-Sachs Disease

- Deficiency of hexosaminidase A
  - Breaks down GM2 ganglioside
- Accumulation of GM2 ganglioside
- More common among **Ashkenazi Jewish** population

Tay-Sachs Disease

- Most common form presents 3-6 months of age
- Progressive neurodegeneration
  - Slow development
  - **Weakness**
  - Exaggerated startle reaction
  - Progresses to **seizures, vision/hearing loss, paralysis**
  - Usually death in childhood
- Cherry red spot
  - No hepatosplenomegaly (contrast with Niemann-Pick)
- Classic path finding: lysosomes with **onion skinning**

Tay-Sachs Disease

- Classic presentation:
  - 3-6 month old infant
  - Ashkenazi Jewish descent
  - Developmental delay
  - Exaggerated startle response
  - Cherry Red spot

Deficiency of hexosaminidase A
Accumulation of GM2 ganglioside

Sulfatides

- Galactocerebroside + sulfuric acid
- Major component of **myelin**
- Broken down by arylsulfatase A
- Metachromatic leukodystrophy
  - Deficiency of arylsulfatase A
  - Accumulation of sulfatides

Metachromatic leukodystrophy

- Autosomal recessive
- Childhood to adult onset based on subtype
  - Most common type presents ~ 2 years of age
  - Contrast with Krabbe's: present < 6 months
- Ataxia: Gait problems; falls
- Hypotonia: Speech problems
- Dementia can develop
- Most children do not survive childhood

Sphingolipidoses

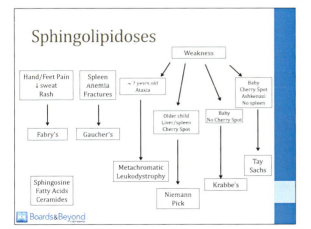

Glycosaminoglycans

- Also called mucopolysaccharides
- Long polysaccharides
- Repeating disaccharide units
- An amino sugar and an uronic acid

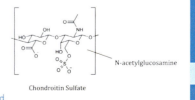

Chondroitin Sulfate

Glycosaminoglycans

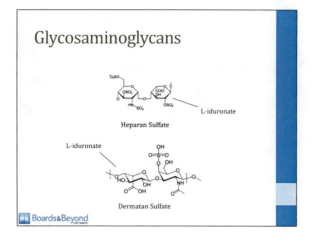

Heparan Sulfate — L-iduronate

Dermatan Sulfate — L-iduronate

Hurler's and Hunter's

- Metabolic disorders
- Inability to breakdown heparan and dermatan
- Diagnosis: mucopolysaccharides in urine
- Types of mucopolysaccharidosis
  - Hurler's: Type I
  - Hunter's: Type II
  - Total of 7 types

Hurler's Syndrome

- Autosomal recessive
- Deficiency of **α-L-iduronidase**
- Accumulation of **heparan and dermatan sulfate**
- Symptoms usually in 1st year of life
- Facial abnormalities ("coarse" features)
- Short stature
- Intellectual disability
- Hepatosplenomegaly

Dysostosis Multiplex

- Radiographic findings in Hurler's
- Enlarged skull
- Abnormal ribs, spine

Hurler's Syndrome

- **Corneal clouding**
  - Abnormal size arrangement of collagen fibers
- Ear, sinus, pulmonary **infections**
  - Thick secretions
- Airway obstruction and sleep apnea
  - Tracheal cartilage abnormalities

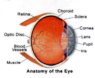

Anatomy of the Eye
BruceBlaus/Wikipedia

Hunter's Syndrome

- X-linked recessive
- Deficiency of **iduronate 2-sulfatase** (IDS)
- Similar to Hurler's except:
  - Later onset (1-2years)
  - No corneal clouding
  - Behavioral problems
  - Learning difficulty
  - Trouble sitting still (can mimic ADHD)
  - Often aggressive behavior

I-cell Disease
Inclusion Cell Disease

- Subtype of **mucolipidosis** disorders
  - Combined features of sphingolipid and mucopolysaccharide
- Named for inclusions on light microscopy
- Similar to Hurler's
  - Onset in 1st year of life (some features present at birth)
  - Growth failure
  - Coarse facial features
  - Hypotonia/Motor delay
  - Frequent respiratory infections
  - Clouded corneas
  - Joint abnormalities
  - Dysostosis multiplex

I-cell Disease
Inclusion Cell Disease

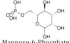
Mannose-6-Phosphate

- Lysosomal enzymes synthesized normally
- Failure of processing in **Golgi** apparatus
  - **Mannose-6-phosphate** NOT added to lysosome proteins
  - M6P directs enzymes to lysosome
  - Result: enzymes secreted outside of cell
- Key findings:
  - Deficient intracellular enzyme levels (WBCs, fibroblasts)
  - Increased extracellular enzyme levels (plasma)
  - **Multiple** enzymes abnormal
  - Intracellular **inclusions** in lymphocytes and fibroblasts

Pompe's Disease
Glycogen Storage Disease Type II

- Acid alpha-glucosidase deficiency
  - Also "lysosomal acid maltase"
- Accumulation of glycogen in lysosomes
- Classic form presents in infancy
- Severe disease → often death in infancy/childhood

Made in United States
North Haven, CT
02 May 2023